W9-AVY-609

ROLE OF THE NURSE IN MANAGED CARE

Lanis L. Hicks, Ph.D.
Janet M. Stallmeyer, R.N., M.S.N.
John R. Coleman, Ph.D.

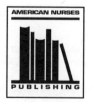

American Nurses Publishing is the publishing program of
the American Nurses Foundation,
an affiliate organization of the American Nurses Association.

Key contributions to the preparation of *The Role of the Nurse in Managed Care* were made by the National Center for Managed Health Care Administration at the University of Missouri (Kansas City and Columbia campuses), and the Group Health Association of America. Publication of this book would not have been possible without their assistance.

Printing and distribution of this book were made possible by a grant from Marion Merrell Dow, Inc.

ISBN 1-55810-086-5
Published by
American Nurses Publishing
600 Maryland Avenue, SW
Suite 100 West
Washington, DC 20024-2571

TABLE OF CONTENTS

PREFACE

The purpose of this material is to discuss the various roles of the nurse in managed care. The materials are presented in three major sections. The first section provides an introductory overview of the role of managed care in the health care delivery system. In this section, the concept of managed care is defined, historical trends are described, and alternative organizational structures are discussed. In addition, various types of provider controls and authorization systems are described and their implications discussed.

In the second section, various roles for the nurse in managed care are defined. While the roles described in this section are not exhaustive, they do demonstrate the wide scope of functions and activities nurses perform in managed care organizations. In general, these roles encompass the provision of health care services, patient advocacy, and the management of resources. Within each specific topic, the function or activity is defined and the role of the nurse is discussed. Finally, illustrations of how nurses have performed various functions or activities within managed care are provided.

The third section discusses the future of managed care and nursing. As the changes in the health care system lead to convergence of the futures of managed care and nursing, nurses must take the initiative in meeting the challenges associated with this convergence. Internally, nurses must seize the current opportunities to become intrapreneurs in assisting their organizations adapt to the changing environments in order to meet the needs of their clients and to increase professional growth and satisfaction. Externally, nurses are faced with many new opportunities to become entrepreneurs in providing services to managed care organizations in meeting the needs of their clients and increasing their professional growth and development. The education and philosophy of nursing places nurses in an excellent position to move the managed care organizations from a paradigm of medicine to a paradigm of health.

SECTION ONE

OVERVIEW OF MANAGED CARE

What is *managed care?* There is no single, uniformly accepted descriptor of an organizational structure that defines managed care. Instead, the term has been applied to a wide variety of "prepayment arrangements, negotiated discounts, and agreements for prior authorizations and audits of performance" (Madison and Konrad 1988, 250). As this definition indicates, managed care spans a broad continuum of entities, from the simple requirement of prior authorization for a service in an indemnity health insurance plan to the assumption of all legal, financial, and organizational risks for the provision of a set of comprehensive benefits to a defined population.

A common thread running through all these variations in managed care, however, is that some type of restriction on traditional fee-for-service medicine's unlimited access to providers who are paid on a usual, customary, and reasonable charge basis is introduced into the decisions made by consumers and providers under some type of binding contract arrangement. The purpose of these restrictions is to modify the behaviors of providers and consumers through financial penalties and rewards and through delivery mechanism controls to improve the efficiency of the health care delivery system. The goal of a managed care system, therefore, is to get the decision makers (providers, consumers, payers) to consider carefully the relative efficacy and importance of various services, procedures, and treatment modalities and to make decisions regarding the allocation of their limited resources accordingly (Langwell 1990). The goal of managed care is not simply to lower costs but, also, to ensure that maximum value is received from the resources used in the production and delivery of health care services to the population.

Definitions

Health Maintenance Organizations

While the generic term managed care encompasses a wide variety of organizational structures, these organizations can be categorized into three basic types: *health maintenance organizations* (HMOs), *preferred provider organizations* (PPOs), and *private managed indemnity* health insurance plans (Curtiss 1990). The most structured and controlled type of managed care arrangement is the health maintenance organization, a term coined by Paul Elwood in 1970 to emphasize the positive health promotion focus of this health care structure (Davis et al. 1990). Like the term managed care, the term health maintenance organization is a generic covering a wide array of organizational structures. In general, however, HMOs are distinguished from traditional fee-for-service health care systems by having the common characteristic of combining the delivery and financing of health care services into one organized system.

In general, HMOs include the following five features (Luft et al. 1980):

1. The HMO assumes an explicit contractual responsibility for providing a stated range of health care services.
2. There is an enrolled, defined population.
3. Subscribers voluntarily enroll in the plan and providers voluntarily participate in it.
4. The HMO receives a fixed periodic payment (a capitation rate per enrollee) from the subscribers, which is established independently of actual utilization by an individual subscriber.
5. The HMO assumes financial risk for the contracted services.

These five behavioral features broadly define the distinguishing characteristics of HMOs. As these features indicate, HMOs combine utilization management, provider selection, and financial incentives to modify or control the behavior of providers in the system. Although other entities use some of these tools, HMOs are unique in the inclusion of *all* these features in their organizations (Langwell 1990).

Traditionally, enrolled members of HMOs were financially covered for health services only if they received those services from providers participating in the plan or if these participating providers pre-authorized the member to receive certain services from a designated provider outside the plan. These site-of-service restrictions on consumers' freedom to choose providers at the time of the consumption of services enabled the HMO to control utilization and to improve efficiency of medical service delivery. By controlling where consumers can obtain services, HMOs can coordinate access to the appropriate type of service more effectively.

While these site-of-service restrictions are important to the HMO's ability to achieve appropriate utilization, efficiency, and effectiveness, they are usually the features consumers find to be the most onerous. Consumers of health care services often desire greater freedom in their ability to select a provider from whom to receive a particular service

(Boland 1991). In response to this desire for increased freedom of choice, two relatively new organizational structures have evolved—PPOs and a derivative of traditional HMOs called *point-of-service* (POS) products or options. In addition, indemnity insurance plans are moving from simply offering passive risk-sharing arrangements to taking an active role in managing provider and member utilization of the services they cover (Boland 1991). This change by indemnity health insurance plans is narrowing the distinctions among traditional insurance and the various forms of managed care.

Preferred Provider Organizations

The term preferred provider organization does not describe a single type of arrangement or have a single definition. Instead, it is a generic term referring to a variety of arrangements. In general, these arrangements fall somewhere between a traditional HMO and a standard indemnity health insurance plan, and usually include some characteristics of both.

One of the primary distinguishing characteristics of a PPO is its structural design which provides financial incentives rather than controls to enrolled members to persuade them to prefer to receive their necessary health care services from a member of a designated select panel of health care providers. (Usually these incentives include waiver of deductibles—a flat amount consumers must pay before the insurance coverage pays anything—and reductions in coinsurance requirements—a percent of the price of services for which the consumer retains responsibility). Ideally, the providers on this preferred panel have been selected to participate on the basis of their cost-efficiency, quality, and effective practice management. Other common characteristics of preferred provider organizations are (Gannon 1985):

1. The panel of providers may include hospitals, physicians, and other health professionals.
2. The PPO business functions and marketing activities are centralized, but the provider management process is decentralized.
3. The PPO provides a utilization review program with supporting cost control information.
4. In return for more prompt payment of claims submitted, providers accept a negotiated discount PPO fee as payment in full and do not bill patients for additional amounts.
5. The establishment of selective conditions for provider participation, theoretically, allows the organization to eliminate ineffective and inefficient providers from the panel of preferred providers.

6. The panel of participating providers maintains independent medical practices, enabling its members to continue to treat their private patients as well as PPO members.

While the specific elements included in PPOs may vary in restrictiveness, an underlying concept in all types of these arrangements is the expectation that the concessions made by the participants in the arrangement will be more than offset by the financial advantages accruing to them (Palmer 1985). PPOs reward patients through financial incentives for using a select panel of providers and reward providers for practicing conservative medicine by including them on the list of preferred providers. The PPO contracts with providers for discounted prices and utilization review activities before the patient enters the system, not just retrospectively. This feature of prior negotiations establishes more well-defined and better understood boundaries for the operation of the health care system. As in any other activity, participants tend to perform better when the rules of the game are explicitly stated up front.

In general, PPO providers do not assume an insurance risk; that risk is assumed by a third party. The providers may, however, assume substantial business risk in terms of the negotiated fees they agree to accept. If the increased number of patients generated by the PPO is not sufficient to overcome the reduction in the fees previously charged, the provider may experience a reduction in income by participating in the arrangement. Since most PPO providers are paid on a discounted fee-for-services basis, and therefore do not bear the financial risk for excessive utilization of their services, it is essential that the PPO arrangement contain effective utilization review programs to keep providers from inducing increases in volume and complexity of services to compensate for the reduced price (Gabel and Ermann 1985). Otherwise, the PPO may not be able to achieve its anticipated cost savings for the system as providers alter their practice patterns in an undesired direction.

In joining a PPO, consumers are encouraged—through financial incentives to reduce out-of-pocket costs—to utilize a select panel of providers. However, unlike members of HMOs, PPO members do not lose all financial coverage of health care services if they elect to go outside the panel of approved providers for their health care services; their standard indemnity insurance coverage with deductibles and coinsurance amounts is still in effect. This feature enables consumers to exercise freedom of choice in selecting a provider each time they interact with the health care system, not just when they initially select their health insurance plan (Jones 1990). This option is very appealing to many people because they can select a provider on the panel for one type of service and a nonparticipating provider for another; or they can see a participating provider one time for a particular problem and elect to see a nonparticipating provider the next time. Consumers are not financially "locked in" to a specific set of providers when they participate in a PPO arrangement.

Because of the wide diversity of forms and the rapidity with which PPOs are evolving, it is very difficult to conduct an empirical analysis of their full impact (Tibbitts and Manzano 1984). One thing that is happening, however, as various payers attempt to control costs, is that providers have less opportunity to shift the costs of uncompensated care to other payers, reducing their ability to provide services to individuals who are unable to pay. This reduction in cost-shifting ability is increasing the need to address explicitly the issues raised by the 31 million uninsured Americans (Health Insurance Association of America 1990).

Traditional Health Insurance

The traditional indemnity health-insurance plans offer two types of coverage—cost of services utilized or pre-established cash amounts for services utilized. Under a cost-of-services indemnity plan, such as that originally used by Blue Cross and Blue Shield, the insurance carrier provides financial protection against all costs associated with a covered service (e.g., thirty days of hospital care), exclusive of deductibles and coinsurance (Kongstvedt 1989). The consumer, therefore, has no incentive to shop around for the most cost-effective provider because the insurance carrier has agreed to provide total financial coverage for a service—regardless of the unit price or total cost of the service—up to the maximum amount of service allowed by the policy.

Under a cash indemnity plan, such as that originally used by most private insurance companies, the insurance carrier provides financial coverage for a service—up to a pre-established amount, to be applied toward the cost of a covered service (e.g., $500 per day for hospital care)—exclusive of deductibles and coinsurance (Kongstvedt 1989). The consumer has only an incentive to select a provider under the designated limit, not necessarily select the most cost-effective provider. The consumer also has to keep modifying the policy to maintain adequate coverage in the inflationary health-care system.

Under indemnity health-insurance plans, the emphasis is on financing health care services, and the provision of services is only tangentially considered. In most instances, it is the sole responsibility of the subscriber to identify the need for care and to locate a provider of such care (Shouldice and Shouldice 1990). In addition, most indemnity insurance plans historically covered only selective services or sites of care and did not provide comprehensive health-care coverage. For example, most plans covered services (physicals, tests, surgical procedures, treatments) if they were provided on an inpatient basis by hospitals but did not pay for the same services if they were performed in a physician's office or on an ambulatory basis. Consequently, this type of coverage caused an overuse of services in the covered location relative to other sources of care (Feldstein 1988).

Under most service indemnity types of health insurance plans, the providers contractually agree to accept a negotiated payment schedule for services provided to subscribers of the plan, and payment for services usually is made directly to the provider rather than to the subscriber. Under cash indemnity health-insurance plans, the subscriber often has to pay for services at the time of receipt and then receive reimbursement from the insurance company, unless the provider agrees to accept assignment of payment from the insurance carrier and bill the patient for the balance (Curtiss 1990).

Historically, the indemnity insurance industry functioned as a passive risk-sharing system, paying whatever providers requested and passing the expenses on to purchasers in the form of higher premiums. As the indemnity health-insurance industry evolved, it incorporated into its structure such inflationary features as "free choice of providers, cost- and charge-based reimbursement, fee-for-service payment, and differential subsidies favoring inpatient hospital care" (Higgins and Meyers 1986, 3).

As cost containment pressures have risen and indemnity insurance plans have experienced increased competition from alternatives, they also have introduced a variety of new techniques into their structures— e.g., preadmission screening, prior admission approval, second opinions for surgery, continued stay certification, retrospective review, and discharge planning. These techniques are directed at managing utilization of health care services and thereby moderating the rate of increase in the costs of their programs. As indemnity insurance carriers introduce more restrictions on their beneficiaries' utilization of services, the distinctions between the indemnity insurance industry and the formal managed-care industry become very blurred.

Point-of-Service Option

Another feature blurring the distinction between indemnity insurance and managed care is the "point-of-service" option currently being adopted by many traditional HMOs. Under this new feature, enrolled members of HMOs are allowed to select a nonparticipating provider each time they need a service, and to do so without adhering to the HMO's standard protocol for out-of-plan use. This point-of-service option enables the enrolled members to receive coverage for the services utilized out-of-plan. In return for this increased freedom of choice, enrolled members usually pay substantially higher costs in terms of increased premiums, deductibles, and coinsurance if they select a provider outside the HMO panel of participating providers (Curtiss 1990).

These increased costs are designed to compensate the HMO for its reduction in control over its members' utilization of health care services and for the potentially higher-cost providers selected by the members (Curtiss 1990). The increased freedom of choice permitted by this feature addresses the concerns many individuals and employers have of being locked in to specific providers for their health care services. However, there are costs associated with the reduction in control exercised by HMOs, and these costs must be borne by the enrolled participants.

Role In The Health Care System

Rising Expenditures

Both public and private expenditures for health care services in the United States have been increasing. Total expenditures from all sources increased from $249.1 billion in 1980 to $604.1 billion in 1989. During this period, health care expenditures rose from $1,059 to $2,354 per capita, and the percentage of gross national product (GNP) represented by the health care sector increased from 9.1 percent to 11.6 percent. In 1989, Medicare financed 17 percent of health care expenses, Medicaid 10 percent, other governmental programs 15 percent, private health insurance 33 percent, and other private sources 4 percent. Consumers financed only 21 percent of total health expenditures out of pocket (Levit et al. 1991).

As the rate of increase in health-care expenditures has accelerated in recent years, increasing at a rate of 11.9 percent during 1989, so have pressures to control health care costs. The data in Table 1 provide a general overview of the rate of growth in health care expenditures between 1960 and 1989. The first set of expenditures data indicates the total amount spent on health care in billions of dollars; the second set

Table 1: **U.S. Health Expenditures**

Year	$ Billions	Per Capita	% of GNP
1960	$ 27.1	143	5.3
1965	41.6	204	5.9
1970	74.4	346	7.3
1975	132.9	592	8.3
1980	249.1	1,059	9.1
1985	420.1	1,700	10.5
1989	604.1	2,354	11.6

Source: Lazenby and Letsch, 1990.

indicates the average amount spent per person on health care services; and the third set indicates the percent of GNP accounted for by the health care industry.

Management of Care

As employers, governments, payers, consumers, and providers increasingly seek methods for containing the rate of increase in health care costs while continuing to ensure access to necessary, high-quality health care services, more and more emphasis will be placed on "managing" the utilization and production of health care services. Through the use of techniques such as selective contracting, utilization review, pre-authorization, and risk-sharing with providers, and through the use of primary care providers (primary care physicians, nurse practitioners, and physician assistants) as controllers of access to the system, utilization and therefore costs can be controlled more effectively. As these techniques illustrate, the basic premise of managing care is to place incentives or restrictions (internal or external) on the decisions made by providers and consumers to ensure that the benefits of an encounter or service are considered relative to the costs. As pressures increase requiring justification from providers, payers, and consumers for rising expenditures on health services, all participants in the health care system will find it necessary to improve the effectiveness and efficiency of the resources used in the production and consumption of health care services.

The emphasis on containing costs by managing the utilization of health care services is not without danger, however. Whereas the traditional health-care financing and delivery systems often had adverse incentives for the overutilization of services, especially resource-intensive services such as hospital care, managed care has the potential for creating incentives for the under-utilization of services and resources and for unduly limiting access to necessary and appropriate health-care services. Consequently, as more and more providers are forced to adopt various strategies for managing the care provided to their patients, mechanisms must also be put in place for monitoring the quality of care provided and for ensuring the population's access to appropriate health-care services (Chambers 1990).

In the last few years, managed health care is no longer being referred to as an alternative health-delivery system; it has instead become accepted as a vital part of mainstream medicine. This acceptance has occurred rapidly as all facets of the health care system have been forced to implement various strategies to control health care costs.

As efforts to control costs intensify, providers increasingly will be asked to assume the financial risks associated with treating their patients and, as a result, will adopt practices to manage the care provided to their patients. This assumption of financial risk by the provider gives professionals an incentive to be cognizant of the relative prices of the resources they use and to use them more efficiently and effectively (Chambers 1990). Professional ethics, personal integrity, and outside controls will all be necessary to ensure that everyone has access to appropriate health-care services in this new, constrained health-care environment.

Key Focus

As the management of health care services intensifies, patient access to a system of comprehensive and coordinated services increasingly will be focused on a single entry point into the system. The ability of patients to decide unilaterally to access various points of entry will be dramatically curtailed, if not eliminated, and access will be coordinated through a single unit designated by the entity that is at financial risk for the utilization of services.

Historical Trends

Although organizations providing comprehensive services for a predetermined fee (prepaid group practices) have been around since the eighteenth century, systematic data collection was sparse until the early 1970s. In 1973, P.L. 93–222 was passed, authorizing the expenditure of federal funds for the establishment and development of HMOs. To become qualified for federal funding, HMOs were required to provide a prescribed range of rather comprehensive basic health services and additionally to offer an extensive set of optional services that prescribers could purchase through the HMO. In addition, the initial act required HMOs to use community ratings in establishing premiums rather than experience ratings and to offer a period of open enrollment during which anyone could join. Another feature of the original act, referred to as the dual choice requirement, was that employers were required to offer an HMO option to their employees, if a federally qualified HMO was available in the area. "A number of amendments have been made to the HMO Act of 1973, the most important of which are the elimination of the specific list of optional supplemental health care services that must be offered and the modification of the community rating system to allow HMOs to community rate by class" (Langwell 1990, 74).

Health Maintenance Organizations

Whereas growth in the number of prepaid health plans or HMOs and in the number of people enrolled in these organizations was slug-

Figure 1: **Growth in HMO Plans**

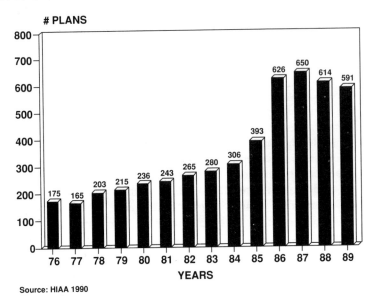

Source: HIAA 1990

gish prior to 1970, growth has been very rapid during the past two decades. In 1970, there were 37 HMOs in the United States, enrolling less than 2 million members. In 1989, there were 591 health maintenance organizations in operation and enrollment was almost 35 million. In 1989, more than 13 percent of the population in the United States was enrolled in HMOs, with only two states (Alaska and Mississippi) not offering plans available to their residents (HIAA 1990). Growth in enrollment in HMOs is still occurring, although at a slower rate than in the mid-1980s because of increased availability of competing organizations and the difficulty HMOs encounter in offering employers experience-rated premiums (Gruber, Shadler, and Polich 1988). Figure 1 shows the trend in the number of HMO plans in existence in the United States between 1976 and 1989 and Figure 2 shows the increase in members enrolled in HMOs between 1976 and 1989.

As the data in Figure 1 indicate, the number of HMO plans peaked at 650 in 1987 and then declined to 614 in 1988, and declined further to 591 in 1989. Much of the decline in numbers of plans was a result of mergers and acquisitions within the industry.

Another trend, and one not reflected in the above data, has been the conversion of tax-exempt (nonprofit) HMOs to investor-owned (for-profit or proprietary) status. In addition to a substantial number of existing tax-exempt HMOs converting to investor-owned status, a large majority of the new HMOs entering the market are doing so as investor-owned entities. As a result, the majority of HMOs currently in the market are investor-owned (Langwell 1990).

Houck and Mueller (1988) suggested that the historical prohibition against the corporate practice of medicine and the availability of federal funds only to tax-exempt organizations may have been largely responsible for the early emphasis on the tax-exempt form of organizations. As federal funds for development and start-up of HMOs became generally unavailable over time, both state and federal restrictions on the operations of investor-owned entities subsided and the restrictions on the amount of debt that not-for-profit HMOs could issue, the increased access to equity capital markets, and the greater ability to diversify available to investor-owned entities encouraged the move to this form of organization. In addition, under recent interpretations the Internal Revenue Service has held that HMOs cannot act as insurers of health care services (as opposed to deliverers of health services) and still retain their tax-exempt status. All of these organizational and financial factors have combined to increase the attraction of the investor-owned status for HMOs. As a result, HMOs, like many other participants in the health care field, are selecting the investor-owned mode of organization.

As the data in Figure 2 indicate, the number of members enrolled in HMOs has been steadily increasing. In 1976, there were only 6 million people enrolled in HMOs; in 1989, that number had risen tremendously, to 34.7 million. The most rapid growth in enrollment in HMOs occurred during 1986, when enrollment grew almost 36 percent. During 1989, enrollment in HMOs increased at the modest rate of slightly over 6 percent.

HMOs have appeal as a cost containment strategy because of the incentives they give providers to be more efficient in their use of resources in rendering services to their patients. Evidence (Harris and Associates 1984; Luft 1978; Taylor and Kagay 1986) has shown that when total costs (premiums plus out-of-pocket expenditures) are compared, HMOs do have lower costs than traditional fee-for-service plans. However, although costs are lower, there is no evidence (Gruber, Shadler, and Polich 1988; Luft 1980) that the rate at which costs are increasing is any slower in HMOs than in traditional indemnity insurance plans; consequently, the problem of escalating health care costs may not be solved simply with the development of additional HMOs.

Figure 2: **Growth in HMO Enrollment**

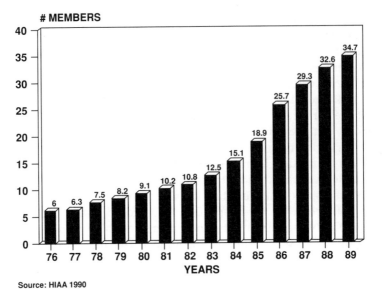

Source: HIAA 1990

Preferred Provider Organizations

PPOs, a relatively new phenomenon that developed in the health care delivery system during the 1980s, are also growing rapidly as an organizational form of medical practice. In 1987, there were 572 PPOs in the United States; by 1989, that number had increased 19.8 percent to 685. In 1988, participation was 36 million, exceeding the number of members enrolled in HMOs (HIAA 1990).

PPOs offer consumers a financial incentive (waived or lower deductibles and coinsurance) to select a specific set of providers when services are needed but allow the freedom to choose each time a service is needed whether to seek services from a participating provider or not. There are no disincentives for participating in an available PPO since coverage of nonparticipating providers is the same in each instance. Currently, data are not available on the impact that PPOs have had on the utilization patterns of consumers, the practice patterns of providers, or on the provider-selection decisions of consumers.

Summary

Currently, almost all traditional indemnity health insurance plans incorporate one or more techniques for managing the utilization of health care services by their subscribers. As more and more traditional indemnity health insurance plans adopt the utilization management features proven to be successful in other types of financing systems, the distinctions among the various forms of financing health care services will become increasingly blurred, making comparative analyses among the various forms even more difficult.

Structure of HMOs

As the HMO industry matured, the distinctions among the various types of health maintenance organizations narrowed dramatically. In response to mounting competitive pressures, mergers, and acquisitions, the mutually exclusive mechanisms that HMOs had used in financing and delivering health services have become blurred; many HMOs now combine several different model types under their umbrella organization. However, the four basic types of HMOs —staff, group, network, and independent practice association—still form a relevant framework for analyzing their structure, incentives, and performance. In general, the distinguishing features of these four categories of HMOs reflect how the HMO relates to its physicians in terms of organization and payment.

Staff Model

In the staff model HMO, "participating physicians are salaried employees of the HMO who provide most outpatient services at the plan's multi-specialty ambulatory care center or centers. Only rarely do these physicians provide a significant volume of fee-for-service care, and any resulting income accrues to the HMO rather than to individual physicians" (Fox and Heinen 1987, 8). This type of plan is the most centrally controlled as services are provided at HMO-owned facilities by employed physicians. As a result, the staff model HMO offers the greatest potential for controlling utilization and costs. An example of the staff model HMO is the Group Health Plan of Puget Sound in Seattle, Washington.

While the organizational entity in the staff model HMO is financially at risk for keeping costs below the capitation premium received, the physicians in the plan are not personally at financial risk for the services because they provide because they are salaried employees. As a result, this type of HMO requires the most management and internal controls to maintain cost efficiency in its operation. To encourage physicians to be cognizant of the relative costs of various resources, treatment modalities, and services, most staff model HMOs must rely heavily on formal utilization controls because they have only limited flexibility in providing financial incentives by allowing physicians to participate in some form of bonus or incentive plan. Under these plans, physicians may earn extra income based on either their individual performance or productivity or on the overall performance of the organization.

Historically, staff model arrangements have been able to provide services to their members at a substantially lower cost than has the traditional fee-for-service method of delivering health care services, mainly through a significant reduction in the utilization of inpatient hospital days. Greenberg and Rodburg (1971) suggested that these savings can be attributed to the following three major factors.

First, staff model HMOs generally provide a comprehensive set of inpatient and outpatient services for their enrollees, whereas traditional fee-for-service insurance programs emphasize hospital and surgical expenses. The coverage of service regardless of site of delivery (inpatient or outpatient) removes the economic incentive to utilize only the site where the service is covered by the insurance policy. This historical advantage will be sharply reduced as other types of insurance plans expand their coverage to non-hospital based services and attach penalties for the utilization of inpatient services when outpatient services are medically appropriate.

Second, under a comprehensive prepayment system that owns its own hospitals or has capitated contractual arrangements with hospitals, the fiscal solvency of the hospital is not increased with increased occupancy since revenues received by the hospital are unrelated to the rate of use. Consequently, it takes fewer beds to service a specific population under this type of arrangement. In addition, since physicians are paid a prenegotiated salary under this type of plan, their incomes are not positively correlated with the amount of services provided, giving them an incentive to practice conservative rather than elaborate medicine.

Third, since the total resources available to the organization are fixed by the prenegotiated rate received per enrolled member, there is an incentive for the organization to control, often through incentive and bonus plans, the physicians' use of resource intensive services, such as hospitals. Under this type of arrangement, the more resources that go for the provision of hospital services, the less that are available for the organization to distribute among physicians.

Although it has been hypothesized that the financial incentives created by the staff model HMO mechanism may exert adverse pressures for providers to overeconomize in the provision of necessary services, evidence (Brook and Kosecoff 1988) comparing the end results of the services provided by the traditional system and the staff model HMO does not identify any discrepancies in outcomes. Greenberg and Rodburg (1971) suggested that, in general, three factors will keep such service erosion within HMOs from occurring.

First, the threat of malpractice in HMOs is just as strong as it is in the traditional fee-for-service practice of medicine. This threat keeps all providers practicing defensive medicine. It has been hypothesized that the staff model HMO may in fact improve the quality of care since the comprehensiveness of the services provided within the plan decreases the provision of episodic care often associated with fee-for-service medicine.

Second, the physicians practicing in the HMO are economically and professionally dependent on the financial stability of the umbrella organization. The economic viability of the organization in turn is very dependent on the continued enrollment of its subscribers; consequently, the physicians cannot risk the members becoming dissatisfied and disenrolling from the plan. As a result, physicians who are asked to join the staff model HMO are carefully screened and are often required to be board certified or board eligible before being accepted into the practice. Efforts are also made to ensure that the physicians practicing in the plan do not have a style of practice that might increase the need for expensive compensatory services.

Third, the peer review pressures exerted by other physicians in the plan, forcing compliance with strict professional norms of good medical care, are probably the strongest disincentive against excessive economizing by physicians. The reputation of all physicians associated with the staff model HMO is based on the overall reputation of the HMO. In addition, because of increased convenience of a unitary medical record and the reduction of financial and distance barriers, increased referrals and consultations among physicians are stimulated.

In addition to the economic incentives created by the staff model mechanism, this arrangement entails certain other advantages (Greenberg and Rodburg 1971). Because of the centralized organizational structure, the staff model HMO enables greater control to be exercised over the utilization of its facilities, allowing providers to use the most economically appropriate facility in the efficacious treatment of an episode of illness. This ability to exert control over the nature of medical care provided should contribute to a substantial reduction in the costs of services.

The staff model practice provides services to a relatively stable, well-defined population. This characteristic enables the group to plan its facilities for a more estimable population, which contributes significantly to the cost reduction advantage of staff model practices.

The inclusion of a comprehensive set of services within the practice also enables the organization to plan more effectively. The combination of a well-defined population with a comprehensive set of services enables the plan to develop relatively accurate estimations of the potential demand for various levels and types of services. In addition, the incentives created within the staff model plan reward providers for rendering the least resource-intensive level of care consistent with acceptable medical standards (Greenberg and Rodburg 1971).

Group Model HMO

In the group model, physician services are arranged for by contracting with an independent multi-specialty group practice, whose members then become the plan's participating doctors. In some situations, the group practice predated the HMO and served only fee-for-service patients. The HMO pays the group a negotiated capitation, that is, a fixed sum per enrollee per month. Referrals to nonparticipating doctors are usually paid out of the capitation also. In addition, there may be a bonus plan to create an incentive for doctors to control hospital costs (Fox and Heinen 1987, 9).

As the above definition indicates, there are two kinds of group models. First, there are the group model HMOs in which "medical services are delivered in the HMO-owned health center or satellite clinic by physicians who belong to a specially formed but legally separate medical group that only serves the HMO" (Schafer, Olson, and Gocke 1987, iv). The best-known example of this type of plan is a Kaiser-Permanente group where the organized physician group (Permanente) is paid a negotiated monthly capitation by the HMO (Kaiser Foundation Health Plan), and the group then distributes the income to the salaried physicians in the group. In this model, the physicians are generally not allowed to provide services on a fee-for-service basis and, organizationally, it has the same incentives as a staff model HMO.

The second type of group model HMO "contracts with an existing, independent group of physicians to deliver medical care. Usually, an existing multi-specialty group practice adds a prepaid component to its fee-for-service mode, becomes a fee-for-service and a prepaid medical group, and affiliates with or forms an HMO" (Schafer, Olson, and Gocke 1987, iv). In this type of HMO, the physicians in the plan provide both fee-for-service medicine and prepaid medical services at the group's clinic facilities. The physicians in this group are also not prohibited from entering into contracts with more than one HMO.

In this type of group model, the medical group is usually paid a negotiated monthly capitation rate for each subscriber. The group then determines how to distribute this income to the members of the group. "Any one of a number of procedures can be used for such distribution: regular fee-for-service equivalent for HMO patients actually served; fee-for-service less a discount; equal shares of the HMO capitation revenue to all physicians regardless of how many prepaid patients they individually served during the month; or a combination of the above methods" (Schafer, Olson, and Gocke 1987, iv).

As indicated above, a group model HMO involves adding a prepaid component to a single, existing multi-specialty group's fee-for-service practice. The HMO plan has only limited control over the practice patterns of the physicians within the group since the physicians are organized outside the HMO's direct management. As a result, the HMO usually uses incentives rather than controls to influence the behavior patterns of physicians to practice more conservative medicine (Langwell 1990).

To minimize the influence of the adverse incentives present in the historic fee-for-service system (hospitalizing patients for convenience, providing greater amounts of ancillary services, encountering patients more frequently), the individual providers must be required to share the risks of cost overruns with the group (Gaus, Cooper, and Hirschman 1977). The more dependent the group is on the HMO for income, the stronger the incentives are to manage the costs of the care provided. When the costs are spread among all physicians in the group and fee-for-service practices are maintained, the incentive for an individual physician to control utilization is significantly diluted. Economic motivation is a fact of life and physicians are influenced by financial incentives. This does not imply that financial incentives are the only motivating force for physicians, only that financial incentives cannot be totally disregarded in understanding the medical practice decisions made by physicians in the system. Consequently, the use of appropriate financial incentives must be considered when structuring the health care delivery and financing systems.

Network Model

Network models closely resemble group model HMOs, except that the HMO contracts with two or more independent group practices. Each group receives capitation payments from the HMO for enrollees who designate that medical group. Most groups that are part of a network continue to serve fee-for-service patients. Increasingly, the groups in the network are either capitated for hospital as well as physician services or share heavily in the risk, subject to a stop-loss, or maximum liability, beyond which the HMO bears full responsibility (Fox and Heinen 1987, 10). An example of a network model is HMO Colorado, sponsored by Blue Cross in the Denver metropolitan area. As a hybrid form of the group model HMO, the incentives and controls established by the structure of the network model are very similar to those created by the group model, especially the second type. Therefore, the discussion above, about group model HMOs, also applies to the network model.

Independent Practice Association

Under the IPA model, rather than relying upon centralized group practices, the HMO, either directly or through a formally organized physician association, generally contracts with solo practitioners and small, typically single-specialty, groups. These HMOs commonly have large panels of participating physicians whose practice is mostly fee-for-service. Consumers are often attracted by easier access to primary care sites and the wider choice of physicians, which may include their present doctors (Fox and Heinen 1987, 11). This model offers the least amount of direct control over utilization by members and production costs in the physician's practice.

In an IPA model there is a "central administrative core that contracts directly with individual physicians who continue to practice in solo settings in their own offices serving both fee-for-service and prepaid patients. They usually are reimbursed on a discounted fee-for-service basis" (Schafer, Olson, and Gocke 1987, iv).

Within an independent practice association, physicians collectively enter into contractual arrangements with the association that, for a prenegotiated fee, provides a specific set of services to a defined population. Basically, the IPA model is one of decentralization in which an association of physicians (who may even be geographically dispersed) provide services to the HMO population in their private offices. Usually, the physicians in the arrangement do not serve the HMO exclusively, but continue to devote a significant part of their services to their private practice patients (Pennsylvania Medical Care Foundation 1978).

The physicians participating in IPAs are at some financial risk in the event that the income negotiated with the HMO is not large enough to cover the costs of providing the designated services to the enrolled population. However, since the physicians are also receiving a substantial portion of their income from their private fee-for-service patients, a loss from the IPA arrangement would not be as severe as it would be under a prepaid arrangement (Fox and Heinen 1987).

The typical IPA recruits large numbers of physicians who have already established a medical practice in a community, allowing these physicians to continue practicing in their existing facilities. If a potential subscriber has already established a relationship with one of these physicians, the enrollee does not have to change physicians when enrolling in the plan, only the method by which the services are financed.

The organization or association acts as a fiscal and marketing intermediary for the physicians participating in the arrangement, but does not directly control the provider's practice of medicine (Thomas 1980). The IPA model is a rather conservative approach to initiating modifications in the traditional health care system and does not require radical changes in the way in which existing physicians in a community provide services.

An advantage of the IPA model is its ability to incorporate a broad range of physicians across wide geographic areas. The substantial capital investment required to establish a staff-type practice is also avoided by utilizing the existing practicing physicians and their facilities. The IPA model is also less disruptive to the traditional delivery system since reimbursement to physicians can be provided on a prorated fee-for-services basis, a method familiar to physicians (Thomas 1980). This model offers a method by which providers can voluntarily modify certain aspects of the delivery system in reaction to financial incentives while maintaining the traditional fee-for-service structure as the dominant reimbursement mechanism for their practice.

A disadvantage of this arrangement is the relatively small amount of control the plan's administration can exercise over the utilization and production activities of its physician members. In an IPA, the participating physicians usually continue to function in a manner very similar to their previous method of practicing medicine, a style which has been determined to be very inefficient in many respects (Richardson 1980). As a consequence, cost savings achieved may not be substantial under this type of arrangement.

Comparative Statistics

The data presented in Table 2 show 1) the number of managed health care plans classified into each type of organizational structure, and 2) the relative number of people enrolled in each type of managed care plan during 1989. As the data indicate, the most dominant type of HMO in 1989 was the IPA, comprising over 60 percent of all HMO plans and enrolling over 42 percent of all HMO members.

Table 2: **Model Type of HMOs**

Model Type	# of Plans	% of Plans	% of Enrollees
Staff	61	10.3	12.4
Group	80	13.5	29.9
Network	89	15.1	14.9
IPA	361	61.1	42.8
Total	519	100.0	100.0

Source: HIAA 1990

Table 3: **Monthly Premium Costs**

Type of Plan	Premium of Individual	Premium of Family
Indemnity	$119	$268
IPA	108	272
Staff/group	124	261
PPO	119	271

Source: HIAA 1990

The data in Table 3 show the average monthly premium costs for individuals and families for indemnity insurance, HMO, and PPO plans by type of plan for 1989. When comparing the costs associated with various types of insurance plans, it is the consumers' total costs (premiums plus out-of-pocket expenditures) that are relevant. Traditionally, participants in HMOs have had minimal out-of-pocket costs, while participants in PPOs have had reduced deductibles and coinsurance requirements, reducing their out-of-pocket costs. Indemnity insurance plans traditionally have required subscribers to be responsible for at least some of their health care expenditures. In the data reported from a survey conducted by the Health Insurance Association of America (1990), the three major types of health maintenance organizations—staff, group, and network—are combined into a single category, referred to as staff/group in the table.

Summary

The definitions and descriptions presented here of the four major types of HMOs are unique and mutually exclusive; in reality, most HMOs today combine various aspects of the different models. It is very difficult to identify a specific organization in its pure form today. And, as the health care system continues to evolve, the distinctions among the various forms will continue to blur, making it exceedingly difficult to identify the specific impacts attributable to the individual components of utilization management, provider selection, and financial incentives. This blurring of boundaries, however, does not negate the value of understanding the different incentives and structures created by the various forms.

Characteristics of Enrollees

By 1989, over 13 percent of the population was enrolled in HMOs, and an even larger percentage participated in some type of PPO arrangement. While lack of data limits the ability to analyze the characteristics of the population participating in PPOs, the characteristics of the population enrolled in HMOs have been studied for a number of years, often with conflicting conclusions. (See, for example, Andersen and Newman 1973; Berki and Ashcraft 1980; Davis et al. 1990; Feldstein 1988; Luft 1980; Luft and Miller 1988; Taylor and Kagay 1986; Wilensky and Rossiter 1986; Wolinsky 1980.)

Demographics

Because the sociological and demographic characteristics of subscribers influence the utilization of health care services, and because the decision to participate in a HMO is voluntary, it is important to analyze the characteristics of enrollees in evaluating the performance of managed care organizations. The major sociological and demographic characteristics of the population are: attitudes toward illness, beliefs concerning efficacy of medical treatment, age, sex, marital status, family size, age of family members, and occupation.

Based on these characteristics, the population enrolled in HMOs is not demographically representative of the overall population in the United States. According to industry survey (Hodges, Camerlo, and Gold 1990), 47 percent of the total population enrolled in established HMO plans in 1988 were male and 53 percent were female, while 49 percent of the general population were male and 51 percent were female. In addition, 51 percent of all members enrolled in HMOs were age 17 to 44; this age cohort comprised only 43 percent of the total population. Overall, women in the primary childbearing years (17 to 44) comprised over 25 percent of the total HMO population, but comprised less than 22 percent of the general population.

In 1988, 3.2 percent of the population enrolled in HMOs were Medicare beneficiaries, while this population accounted for 13.5 percent of the total population. Also in 1988, Medicaid recipients represented only 3 percent of all HMO enrollees, though they constituted 9.4 percent of the general population.

Adverse Selection

Under the general theory of consumer preference, it is argued (Feldstein 1988) that people who anticipate using a significant amount of health care services will select a prepaid health care arrangement because of the control over costs it offers. Within an HMO plan, individuals usually pay a prenegotiated annual premium to the HMO and the plan assumes responsibility for ensuring that the individual has access to all necessary, specified health care services without paying any, or only limited, additional out-of-pocket expenditures.

On the other hand, people who have good existing relationships with a private physician are less likely to change insurance companies and join an HMO. People who are currently under medical treatment for an existing medical condition also are unlikely to change delivery systems regardless of its financial advantage because of their relationships with their current health care providers (Luft et al. 1980).

Conversely, the lower utilization rate of subscribers in HMOs is used by other researchers (Luft et al. 1980) as evidence that the participants of a prepaid arrangement are relatively healthier than the general population. However, "no consistent or definitive evidence has been reported that proves that individuals who join HMOs are healthier than those who remain in the fee-for-service sector" (Davis et al. 1990, 143). In addition, there do not appear to be any significant differences between the health status of the populations in each setting in terms of either acute or chronic conditions treated under either system (Feldstein 1988).

Utilization

The utilization of services by members enrolled in HMOs is substantially less than the overall utilization of services by the general population. According to an industry survey (Hodges, Camerlo, and Gold 1990), HMO enrollees under the age of 65 used 358 inpatient days per 1,000 enrollees in contrast to the national average of 519 inpatient days per 1,000 people. In addition, HMO enrollees age 65 and over used 1,582 days of inpatient hospital care, compared to a national average of 2,970 days per 1,000 people age 65 and over. Enrollees in HMOs also used physician services at a lower rate—3.8 encounters per person under the age of 65 and 7.2 encounters per person age 65 and over compared to 4.3 and 7.8 encounters, respectively, in the general population.

The data in Table 4 show the differences in utilization among the various types of HMOs and in the general population. As the data indicate, average lengths of stay (ALOS) in hospitals, discharges per 1,000 people, and the number of inpatient days per 1,000 people are substantially less than in the general population.

Table 4: **Utilization of HMOs**

Model Type	Discharges Per 1,000	Inpt. Days/1,000	ALOS
Staff	89.0	437	4.9
Group	95.8	462	4.8
Network	90.2	401	4.6
IPA	91.6	431	4.6
All Plans	91.8	433	4.7
General	127.6	834	6.5

Sources: Group Health Association of America, 1990, and HIAA, 1990

Performance

The factors that influence the self-selection decisions of subscribers have major consequences for the evaluation of the performance of HMOs and on the transferability of the results obtained within this type of arrangement to the general health care delivery system. If lower costs and reductions in the utilization of health care services are not the result of the structure and financing mechanisms of the HMO arrangements, but simply reflect the characteristics of the population enrolling in HMOs, then the reductions achieved may not be sustained when this organizational system is expanded to include a larger portion of the general population. Unless the savings observed in this system can be attributed to the structural and financing characteristics of HMOs, then the adoption of this type of system as the predominant form of health services delivery may simply redistribute costs instead of reducing costs by improving the overall efficiency of production within the health care delivery system (Luft et al. 1980). Additional research is needed into the performance of the industry before definitive conclusions can be reached.

Controls in Managed Care

As mentioned earlier, a common thread running through the various forms of managed care is the placement of restrictions (rewards, penalties, mandates) on providers and consumers to modify their behavior in the production and consumption of health care services. The types of restrictions or controls encountered vary with the form that managed care takes, but in general these restrictions are designed to influence favorably the price of health care services, the site at which they are delivered, or their utilization. The restrictions of managed care can be categorized as: 1) financial incentives; 2) utilization controls; 3) medical management practices; and 4) quality improvement tools. As reflected by these measures, the goal of managed care is not simply to reduce costs, but rather to maximize value, which includes considering quality and access, not just price (Chambers 1990). These four categories are not mutually exclusive; they often overlap and interact.

Financial Incentives

One of the most widely used tools for modifying consumer or provider behavior is financial incentives. This tool is designed to alter behavior by either financially rewarding desired actions or financially penalizing undesired actions.

CONSUMERS. Financial incentives are the major tool of managed care organizations in modifying consumers' behavior in using health care services. With consumers forced to assume responsibility for an increasing share of the rising costs of health care through larger deductibles and coinsurances, they are becoming more price sensitive. This increase in consumers' direct out-of-pocket expenses makes costs relevant at the point of service and can now be used to influence provider selection and site of service decisions for many consumers.

PPOs, in general, offer to reduce or eliminate deductibles and coinsurances if the insurance beneficiary utilizes a preferred or designated provider, allowing consumers to minimize out-of-pocket expenses while retaining their scope of benefits and freedom of choice at the time of service (Tibbitts and Manzano 1984). If the beneficiary does not select a designated provider, then the traditional insurance policy is still in force, requiring the individual to pay out-of-pocket the deductible and coinsurance conditions of the plan. This feature means consumers are at least partially at risk financially for the decisions they make in selecting a provider.

HMOs utilize even stronger financial incentives for consumers. Once an individual has made the choice to enroll in HMO, he or she must receive services from a designated provider under established protocol in order for the costs of that service to be covered by insurance. If the enrollee chooses to receive services outside the HMO, then he or she must pay out-of-pocket all costs associated with that care. This obviously creates a strong financial incentive for the enrollee to utilize the designated providers.

Financial incentives are also used by managed care organizations to ensure that the consumer receives services in the most appropriate, least costly setting. To encourage efficient medical decision making, for example, a PPO plan may pay 100 percent of the costs of a surgical procedure performed on an ambulatory care basis, but pay less than 100 percent if the procedure is performed on an inpatient basis. The consumer, therefore, must absorb at least part of the financial consequences of less prudent medical behavior (Barger, Hillman, and Garland 1985).

Similar types of financial incentives can be utilized through requirements for second opinions, preadmission certification, and preauthorization. If the consumers abide by plan protocol, then financial loss is minimized; if they fail to follow the protocol and utilize services differently, then they face a financial penalty.

PROVIDERS. Managed care organizations also use financial incentives in modifying providers' behavior in the production of cost-effective health care services. "Cost effective providers utilize services judiciously, gauging quantity and intensity of care to the medical service requirements of patients" (Boland 1991, 331). The financial incentives to providers depend on the type of payment mechanism used to reimburse for services provided to the beneficiaries. These payment mechanisms should be structured to reward appropriate reduction in resource use or increased results obtained with current resources and to penalize providers financially for inefficient use of resources. To be effective, the financial incentive should provide a direct relationship between provider behavior and financial compensation.

Payment to Institutions. In establishing financial arrangements with institutions for the provision of services to beneficiaries, managed care organizations use four basic payment mechanisms: discounted billed charges, per diem rates, per admission rates, or capitation (Cobbs 1989). Although the use of *discounted billed charges* creates an incentive for the institution to keep costs of producing individual services below the negotiated rate, it does not create an incentive for the institution to be prudent in the combination of services provided to the beneficiaries. In fact, under this type of payment mechanism, the incentive is for the institution to provide excessive ancillary services and to extend lengths of stay for which payment will be received.

"Under a *per diem payment* [emphasis added] arrangement, the organization is paid a flat daily fee to provide specific health services" (Cobbs 1989, 49). The institution's incentive is to minimize the daily production costs of caring for the beneficiaries and to minimize the use of ancillary services, but this creates an incentive to maximize the number of days of care provided within the institution to each admission. In addition, a uniform per diem rate creates an incentive for institutions to be selective in the type of patient admitted so that the case mix and condition severity of patients admitted are favorable to the institution in terms of daily cost of caring for the patient (Barger, Hillman, and Garland 1985).

Under a *payment per admission* mechanism, the institution receives a fixed price (most commonly either an unadjusted average or adjusted for diagnosis) for each episode of care provided. "Payment per admission serves as an incentive toward efficient hospital behavior because it extends financial rewards to those facilities that deal seriously with the difficult task of controlling length of stay. This form of hospital payment also encourages hospitals and their medical staffs to address the fundamental underlying issue of "hospital" inefficiency, i.e., physician practice patterns" (Barger, Hillman, and Garland 1985, 92). Payment per admission still has the shortcoming of not providing a financial incentive to minimize admissions to the institution; the only way for the institution to generate revenue is for patients to be admitted to the institution.

Of the four methods, *capitation* offers the greatest financial incentive for institutions to provide conservative, cost-efficient inpatient services. In the strictest sense, a capitation payment is a set, all-inclusive unit payment for a defined type of care rendered to insured individuals or subscribers over a specified period of time. It is a minimum, guaranteed unit payment with total payment based on the aggregate number of treated individuals. The capitation rate reflects the cost, volume, severity, and intensity of care provided to a specific insured population. The most common form of capitation is a predetermined monthly sum for each enrollee covered by a contracting plan (Cobbs 1989, 51).

Under a capitated payment system, a financial incentive is created for institutions to minimize not only the production costs associated with providing a specific service, but also to minimize the utilization of services within the institution since the institution receives payment regardless of actual utilization of services. With capitation, increased utilization of health care services means increased costs for the institution, not increased revenues.

Payment to Individual Providers. Managed care organizations also use a variety of mechanisms for paying individual providers. PPOs generally use four basic mechanisms: discounted charges, relative value systems, negotiated fee schedules, and capitation (Cobbs 1989). To these, HMOs add salary and various types of provider risk pools. These payment mechanisms vary in their financial incentives for encouraging efficient practice behavior.

The traditional method of paying professionals has been *fee-for-service*. Under this system, the professional independently establishes a charge for a particular service or procedure and then billed the consumer that amount. Although this payment system creates an incentive for the professional to minimize the production costs associated with a particular service or procedure, it does not create an incentive to minimize the number of services or procedures provided per episode of illness. In fact, the incentive is to provide more services per episode since this will generate more revenue (Held and Reinhardt 1980). Managed care organizations are seeking incentives that will encourage professionals to practice appropriate medicine consistent with the smallest possible *total* costs to their enrollees.

The *discounted charges* mechanism simply pays a lower fee for each service provided, but still maintains the basic incentive structure of the fee-for-service system. "With discounted fee reimbursement, each physician experiences the same recovery from charges, regardless of charge level or number of services performed. Therefore, there is no economic incentive to control charge increases or utilization" (Boland 1991, 336). This system continues to reward the high-cost professional with greater revenue.

The *relative value* system defines the relative worth of one service or procedure to another in terms of resources consumed and effort expended. The fees paid to professionals "are computed by multiplying an assigned relative value unit for each procedure by a conversion factor. The conversion factor, or price multiplier, is set by a payer on the basis of an actuarial analysis of anticipated claims" (Cobbs 1989, 53). This method sets the price per unit but does not encourage prudent utilization of health care services. Unless the unit prices accurately reflect the costs of production, then relative values will be distorted and the mechanism will result in a skewed and inefficient mix of services and procedures.

The incentives created by a *negotiated fee schedule* are similar to those established by the relative value system. "A fee schedule is a list of medical procedures organized to include a procedure number (for example, CPT-4 code), procedure description, and specific fee per procedure. . . . The fees in the schedule usually are a function of claims experience, tempered by subjective evaluations of locale, utilization experience, market competitiveness, and relative relationships" (Cobbs 1989, 54). The basic unit on which payment is made is still fee-for-service. One adaptation that can be made in this system is to weight the relative fees in such a way as to encourage the provision of certain services in specific sites, for example to pay a higher fee for a service performed on an outpatient rather than inpatient basis. Overall utilization of services, however, is not curtailed.

Conceptually, the *capitation* of professionals is similar to the capitation of institutions: The professional is paid a fixed monthly amount per panel member enrolled, regardless of services actually rendered. "Under a full capitation approach, the physician is at risk for all medical services, including referral services and hospitalization. A more limited capitation approach is commonly used for primary care reimbursement by IPA model HMOs or for specialty services such as mental health or vision care" (Boland 1991, 339).

Under a capitation system, professionals have an incentive to minimize the costs they incur in treating patients. In containing costs, they can alter the volume of services they supply as well as the methods they use in providing a service. The incentive in a capitated system is to provide fewer services instead of more services for each episode of illness. Capitated professionals also have an incentive to use the least costly mix of inputs (labor, capital, supplies, equipment) (Held and Reinhardt 1980). Under the full capitation system, professionals have an incentive to utilize the least expensive appropriate site of service since they are financially at risk for the costs of all services utilized by their panel of subscribers.

When professionals are reimbursed on a straight salary basis, none of the incentives created by the traditional fee-for-service system exist. Under a salaried system, there are no direct financial incentives for professionals to alter their practice patterns since they are paid a fixed amount regardless of how they utilize resources. Indirectly, of course, salary increases and bonuses are dependent on the financial profitability of the managed care plan (Fox and Heinen 1987). The degree of impact this indirect incentive has on an individual professional's behavior pattern is closely related to the extent to which the reward reflects individual effort versus group achievement. The more individualized the reward structure, the more influence it will have on behavior.

One way of modifying professional behavior through financial incentives is to establish a "risk pool" by withholding part of the fees, which are then distributed based on performance. The objective of the risk pool is to create an incentive for professionals to control costs and utilization by placing them at financial risk for their decisions. "A physician incentive pool can be described as a lump sum of money acquired over a lengthy period of time, perhaps a year, which is redistributed to providers on the basis of individual or collective efficiency as judged by predefined criteria" (Barger, Hillman, and Garland 1985, 95). While the mechanisms employed to redistribute the pooled resources may vary, the intent is to reward more efficient providers.

One mechanism used to redistribute the money is to compare an individual professional's costs of services in the plan to a predefined target cost and to pay the professional a portion of the savings generated by his or her practice in the plan. If the professional's costs are lower than the target, then he or she receives a portion of that differential, assuming monies are available in the pool. Before monies can be distributed to individual professionals, the expenses associated with professionals exceeding the target rate must be deducted. This avoids the problem of the plan having to pay individual bonuses when, overall, the plan loses money. An assumption inherent in this mechanism is that peer pressure can be effective in controlling the behavior of high-cost providers if the other professionals' financial well-being is affected by those actions.

Another pooling mechanism involves redistributing the designated finances based on the overall performance of the group rather than on the performance of the individual. To the extent that the performance goals of the group are met, then monies are available to be distributed among the members of the group.

For any pooling mechanism to be effective, professionals need to receive periodic information regarding their performance so they can make adjustments in their behavior. A mechanism that provides information only at the end of the full period of operation will not provide the professionals with sufficient information to modify their behavior.

Summary. As the preceding discussion illustrates, the objective of financial incentives is to encourage providers to modify their behavior to achieve cost-effective, high-quality care. In order to reach the preferred outcome, providers' actions are either rewarded or penalized financially.

Utilization Controls

In conjunction with financial incentives, managed care plans usually incorporate some type of mandated utilization controls. Utilization control programs are not unique to HMOs or to PPOs; they have been used by indemnity insurance plans for decades to control subscriber expenses. However, the aggressiveness with which they have been applied and the strength and effectiveness of their controls have increased with the growth of formal managed care organizations (Boland 1991).

"A workable definition of utilization management (UM) is that it is the ability of providers and insurers to control costs and enhance the quality of and access to care for patients through the efficient management and provision of medical services" (Cobbs 1989, 103). As this definition implies, to be most effective the utilization management program must be closely associated with the quality assurance program. PPOs especially have relied heavily on utilization control mechanisms for their survival and profitability since they have not been able to exercise meaningful control over the selection of physicians or to implement tangible, productive incentive systems (Barger, Hillman, and Garland 1985, 103).

According to Cobbs (1989, 103–104), the major **objectives** of a utilization control program are:

1. To provide the data necessary for identifying areas of underutilization, overutilization, and inefficient utilization of resources;
2. To assist providers in identifying and eliminating medically unnecessary services;

3. To measure the aspects of quality assessment that relate to efficiency, effectiveness, timeliness, appropriateness, accessibility, and acceptability of services;
4. To provide the tools necessary to evaluate the impact of cost-containment activities on quality of care and to determine the point at which quality may be compromised;
5. To provide the technical expertise necessary to evaluate diagnostic and/or treatment protocols to ensure that both quality and cost-effectiveness issues are addressed in the evaluations;
6. To create an environment of cooperation among hospitals, physicians, and other providers as common goals and objectives are identified and addressed;
7. To provide the necessary mechanism by which structure and process can be objectively evaluated and change can be instituted;
8. To provide a mechanism for responding to questions related to cost or quality raised by payers;
9. To provide the information necessary to document performance and to provide information to clients, regulators, and others as appropriate.

To achieve these objectives, the responsibilities and authority of the various participants in the system should be clearly delineated. In addition, the procedures for conducting the various components of the utilization management plan should be established in writing and personnel should be trained to perform the procedures effectively and efficiently.

The major components of an effective utilization management plan are: prospective, concurrent, and retrospective utilization review; second opinion mandates; and discharge planning. Most managed care organizations utilize a combination of all of these mechanisms on both an inpatient and an ambulatory basis in their efforts to control utilization and costs.

Prospective utilization review, in the case of inpatient services, is often called preadmission certification because it occurs before the patient is hospitalized. "Preadmission certification is a screening process that filters out those patients for which inpatient services are not required. The intention of this review mechanism is to ensure that those persons hospitalized require the intensive and costly services provided within the walls of acute care institutions" (Barger, Hillman, and Garland 1985, 104). Prospective utilization review is usually applied for three reasons: 1) to determine the medical necessity of the service performed on an inpatient basis; 2) to document the extra risks necessitating inpatient care for services usually performed on an outpatient basis;

and 3) to establish plan coverage for certain procedures, for example, cosmetic surgery (Boland 1991).

Prospective utilization review can also be utilized on an ambulatory care basis. For ambulatory services, prior authorization may be required before a patient can be referred to a specialist or before certain tests (such as, magnetic resonance imaging (MRI)) or procedures (such as, physical therapy) may be performed. Such preauthorization requires the provider to justify specific actions that are outside the range of services normally performed by that type of provider. To be most effective, the preauthorization should be for a single visit at a single site only; if additional referral visits are required or if a second referral is necessary, the request should originate from the primary provider (Kongstvedt 1989). This allows the plan greater control over the utilization of services outside the plan.

A special form of prospective utilization review is the **second-opinion** program. Under most second-opinion programs, before any non-emergency surgery can be performed, the patient is required to obtain the opinion of a second physician regarding the necessity and appropriateness of the proposed procedure. While the second opinion most often supports the decision of the first physician, the assumption is that the initial physician will be more conservative in recommending surgery if he or she knows that the decision will be reviewed by another physician (Barger, Hillman, and Garland 1985). As a result of this more conservative practice of medicine, there should be a reduction in the number of marginal surgical procedures performed in the plan.

Concurrent review consists of three basic components: admission review, length of stay review, and discharge planning. The *admission review* process complements the preadmission certification review in that it reexamines the appropriateness of a hospital admission. The concurrent admission review can also be used to review the types of services and procedures being performed on the patient and the medical regimen prescribed to ensure that services that were not preauthorized are not being used (Boland 1991).

"Concurrent *length of stay review* [emphasis added] is an evaluation and monitoring process which attempts to ensure that a patient's length of stay is the shortest possible but most appropriate for the conditions surrounding the patient's admission" (Barger, Hillman, and Garland 1985, 106). In general, the expected duration is determined and the patient is then assigned an expected length of stay based on diagnosis and demographic characteristics. Once this expected length of stay has been assigned, any continued stay beyond this expected length must be approved before continuation. To be effective, the expected lengths of stay have to be restrictive enough to create pressure for providers to discharge patients as soon as medically appropriate, but not so restrictive that virtually every patient requires recertification (Boland 1991).

Concurrent review can also be used in an ambulatory setting. In this situation, the treatment regimen prescribed for individual patients can be monitored and feedback provided to the physician regarding standards and norms associated with specific diagnoses. This feedback loop can be very effective as an educational tool and as a mechanism for modifying practice patterns.

A special form of concurrent review is *discharge planning*. To be most effective, discharge planning should begin at the time of admission if not before, and should be considered part of the overall treatment regimen of the patient. "This planning includes an estimate of how long the patient will be in the hospital, what the expected outcome will be, whether there will be any special requirements on discharge, and what needs to be facilitated early on" (Kongstvedt 1989, 88). Knowing early on what special services or equipment may be required means that actions can be taken to ensure their availability when needed; therefore, the patient will not end up having to stay in the hospital longer because those special requirements are not available. Another critical part of discharge planning is informing the patient and the patient's family about "when they can expect discharge, how the patient will be feeling, what they might need to prepare for at home, and how follow-up will occur" (Kongstvedt 1989, 88–89). All of these activities will help smooth the patient's transition from the hospital to another site of care. If the patient and the family are not adequately prepared for their responsibilities at discharge, then pressure may be placed on the physician to retain the patient in the hospital, a very expensive substitute for more appropriate sites of care.

"**Retrospective review** [emphasis added] is the process of reviewing medical treatments after the service has been provided" (Cobbs 1989, 110). This mechanism tends to be much more punitive since the provider may be denied payment for services previously rendered and therefore be unable to recover the costs incurred in providing care. If prospective and concurrent review mechanisms are operating effectively, then retrospective review should be minimal. A possible nonpunitive use of retrospective review would be to develop provider profiles, usually based on claims data, to be used for educational purposes (Cobbs 1989).

In summary, the objectives of utilization review programs are to influence and control the practice pattern of providers so that cost-effective, high-quality health care services are provided. In general, these utilization management programs gain their power through their ability to deny payment for services, either before or after the service is rendered. Their objectives can best be met when they are coordinated with well-organized medical management practices and quality assessment programs.

Medical Management Practices

Health care professionals, especially physicians, have historically exhibited significant autonomy and strong control over the practice of medicine. However, changing physicians' behavior is critical to the success of a managed care plan since physicians are, directly and indirectly, responsible for approximately 85 percent of the costs of health care services (Cobbs 1989). The objective of medical management practices therefore is to induce physicians to modify their practice behaviors to practice more economical medicine without sacrificing quality of care. The best method for achieving this objective is to educate providers.

Education. It has been shown that for education strategies to be effective in changing physician behavior, "cost savings must be coupled with demonstrations of adequate quality of care for patients; the visible support of clinical authority figures is critical; practicing physicians must be actively involved in patient care decision making; and concrete evidence of excessive ordering of services must be presented to physicians" (Boland 1991; 373–374). Effective education requires massive amounts of data regarding the physicians' practice profiles. In addition, these data have to be reported back to physicians and other decision makers in a meaningful, understandable, and timely way.

"Providing regular and accurate data about an individual physician's performance, from both a utilization and (for risk/bonus models) an economic standpoint, is vital to changing behavior" (Kongstvedt 1989, 75). Physicians are in a much better position to modify their behavior when they have the information enabling them to compare their performance with that of their peers and with norms and standards that have been established by the profession or by the managed care plan. When physicians can critically examine their practice behavior, they are in a better position to determine if their style of medical practice needs to be changed.

Discipline. When voluntary methods fail to persuade providers to modify their practice patterns to conform to plan norms, then discipline and sanctions may have to be invoked. Discipline is a formal process creating documentation of the problem or concern under consideration. In general, this process identifies the unacceptable behavior, outlines acceptable corrective behavior, and describes the consequences of failure to modify behavior. Formal sanctioning is more drastic and has serious legal implications. If sanctions are applied, then due process protecting the rights and responsibilities of both parties must be followed and carefully documented (Kongstvedt 1989). It must be shown that the actions taken against the professional were not arbitrary or capricious. Sanctions are the final action and it is hoped that physicians will comply with the goals of the plan when such pressures are implemented. The objective of medical management practices, therefore, is to manage the use of resources by providers within the system, rather than to deny payment for services rendered.

Quality Improvement Tools

Quality assurance issues are gaining importance in the health care system, especially as managed care plans grow in importance. According to Boland (1991), there are five forces contributing to the demand for quality controls. First, there is the assumption that cost containment activities (risk contracts, prospective payment, capitated delivery systems) have the potential to impact negatively on the quality of care available. Second, there is growing consumer awareness of the wide range of quality available in the system, which is in conflict with consumers' expectations for certainty and predictability of outcomes from the system. Third, the intense competitiveness among providers are focused on demonstrated quality and value rather than price, and consumers are expecting verification of the claims of higher quality. Fourth, the complexity of medical care and the large number of interactions among various segments of the system increase the demand for an integrated quality assurance system. Fifth, the assumption that quality is directly related to expenditures increases the perceived conflicts between quality and cost containment.

In response to these concerns, those managed care organizations that are multi-specialty medical group practices or prepaid group practice plans may offer the following factors as indicators that the care they provide can be of higher, not lower quality (Shouldice and Shouldice 1990, 255–256):

1. Because of the regular hours, financial advantages, and periodic sabbaticals available to many group physicians, there is both time for and encouragement of continuing education. The doctors in group practices may be expected to be "better" because they will be more aware of new discoveries.
2. Strict quality control is ensured through constant peer review and free exchange of patients among physicians within the group.
3. Patients with complications will be referred to a specialist immediately, as there is no threat to the primary care physician of losing his fee or his patient.

4. Consultation with specialists in one's own group will be easier and faster than referral to an outside specialist.
5. The unit medical record facilitates good continuity of care; every test, X-ray, and diagnosis is recorded and available to each doctor the patient sees within the group. This also prevents costly duplication of tests, and ensures that treatments (especially prescriptions) for two different conditions by two different doctors will not conflict.
6. Preventive medicine is an element of high-quality care, and this is emphasized by prepaid group practice.

As concerns about quality of care increase, the traditional quality assurance programs are no longer adequate to address these concerns. As a result, more comprehensive quality improvement programs for defining, monitoring, and evaluating quality are being implemented. The ability to monitor quality in managed care organizations is especially important because consumers have limited choice at point of service and the plans have incentives to limit utilization of services (Davis et al. 1990). A major problem encountered in monitoring quality is the lack of adequate measures of quality, especially measures of the outcomes associated with health services. As a consequence, the focus of most quality insurance programs has been on the structural measures of quality.

Traditionally, efforts to provide quality health care focused on quality assessment and quality assurance programs. "Quality assessment defines and measures quality of clinical care and focuses almost exclusively on physician functions and activities. It generally defines quality to consist of a technical component (accuracy and effectiveness of diagnosis and treatment) and an interpersonal component (the caring function). Its application involves identifying targets or indicators, setting standards for acceptable performance, and comparing provider performance to specified standards" (Boland 1991, 424). The purpose of such an assessment is to uncover patterns of care within the system that may result in substandard or low-quality care being provided to subscribers within the system.

To be effective, a quality assurance program must be systematic, objective, ongoing, and integrated (England, Patterson, and Glass 1989). The initial steps in analyzing quality are to determine whether the providers within the system are competent and properly credentialed in the areas in which they are providing services and whether the style of medicine practiced is consistent with professionally established standards. The quality of care being provided is assessed by monitoring certain indicators of performance.

An indicator is a measurable variable related to the structure, process, or outcome of care. Structures are inputs into care, such as resources, levels of care, equipment, or numbers and qualifications of staff. Processes of care are those functions carried out by physicians, including assessment, planning of treatment, evaluation of medical indications for procedures and treatments, technical aspects of performing treatments, and management of complications. Outcomes include complications, adverse events, short-term results of specific procedures and treatments, readmissions, and patient long-term health and functional status (Cobbs 1989, 117). To be utilized effectively, these indicators must be well defined and measurable. Thresholds of acceptable performance must be established and deviations from these thresholds must trigger some type of intervention or corrective action.

Quality assurance programs are not nearly as well defined as quality assessment programs, mainly because there is not a good understanding of how changing physician practices relates to quality of care. "Most assurance programs simply consist of educating the professional about good clinical practices. In general, most assurance programs assume surveillance of physicians will create an incentive to conform to a minimum acceptable standard. It suggests that by informing physicians of their shortcomings, they will correct the deficiencies" (Boland 1991, 425).

Currently, attention is focusing on quality improvement strategies that are more comprehensive than the traditional approaches and that incorporate more people in the organization and wider ranges of theories and concepts. The concept gaining the most attention now is quality improvement management, either Total Quality Management (TQM) or Quality Improvement (QI). "The central purpose of quality improvement management theory (QI) is to create organizations with a clear vision of what constitutes quality for their 'customers,' and how every individual working for them contributes to continually improving the quality of their daily work" (Boland 1991, 425). This approach deviates from the traditional quality assessment and quality assurance programs in its emphasis on system analysis and process improvement. In this approach, the health care delivery system is viewed as being composed of a large number of small, interrelated processes, and it is the quality and efficiency achieved in each of these small units that determines the overall quality and efficiency of the organization. Instead of focusing on the quality of the individual performing the activity, the major focus of this approach is on the quality of the process design (Boland 1991).

"A second relevant principle from QI is that in order for an organization to achieve high quality services or production, everyone working in the organization must know who their customers are and understand their needs and expectations. 'Customer' is a generic term referring to dependency in relationships. The customer is the person who depends on a supplier for a product or service" (Boland 1991, 426). As this definition of customer implies, the patient is not the only customer within a managed care organization. The physician is a customer when he or she is dependent on the laboratory to supply test results; the nurse is a customer when he or she is dependent on medical records for information regarding a patient's history. In order to design an effective, high-quality process, it is necessary that everyone know who all the customers are in the system and what expectations and needs each of these customers has. The basic philosophy (Boland 1991) of a quality improvement program is that inspection systems directed at identifying outlier behavior and outcomes are not effective; the focus needs to be on improving the process of delivering care so that individuals in the system are assisted in providing high-quality care.

Future Issues

The organizational and structural boundaries that historically separated managed care plans from traditional indemnity insurance plans have become blurred and the distinctions will continue to decrease as the health care industry continues to face pressures to contain costs. The labels historically assigned are no longer appropriate as managed care plans offer point-of-service options and indemnity insurance plans adopt stricter provider selection criteria, utilization management procedures, and quality improvement protocols.

In the future, internal and external controls increasingly will be adopted by all financing and delivery health care systems. The emphasis increasingly will be on providing high-quality health care in a system that produces cost savings for members and for the employers who pay a significant portion of health insurance premiums.

To meet the challenge facing the managed care industry to control medical-related expenditures, Miller (1989) identified three issues that would have to be addressed:

1. New management and service delivery products will have to be developed that address the areas where earlier such products have been insufficient. Because professional costs are increasing more rapidly than other segments of the health care sector, managed care plans can expect to face even greater pressures to monitor and control physician behavior.
2. Specialization among managed care plans will increase. To improve efficiency and effectiveness—and to be able to offer greater coverage, service, and cost control—managed care plans will identify and contract with "centers of excellence" for pro-

curing the low-volume, high-cost specialty services and selected procedures needed by their enrollees.
3. Better integration of managed care services will need to occur. To be more effective, managed care organizations will need to improve their management and administrative systems to handle the interface among payers, users, and providers.

The service and delivery products offered by managed care organizations in the future will need to be sophisticated and efficient. Not only will these organizations be expected to provide cost-efficient care, they will be expected to document this for their customers. The expectation is that these organizations can manage quality care—not just costs of services—efficiently and effectively.

References

Andersen, R., and J. Newman. 1973. Societal and individual determinants of medical care utilization in the United States. *Milbank Memorial Quarterly* 51(1): 95–124.

Barger, S.B., D.G., Hillman, and H.R. Garland. 1985. *The PPO handbook.* Rockville, MD: Aspen Systems.

Berki, S., and M.L.F. Ashcraft, 1980. "HMO enrollment: Who joins what and why: A review of the literature. *Milbank Memorial Quarterly* 58(4): 588–632.

Boland, P. 1991. *Making managed healthcare work: A practical guide to strategies and solutions.* New York: McGraw-Hill, Inc.

Brook, R.H., and J.B. Kosecoff. 1988. Competition and quality. *Health Affairs* 7(3): 150–161.

Chambers, S.K. 1990. *The insider's guide to managed care: A legal and operational roadmap.* Washington, DC: The National Health Lawyers Association.

Cobbs, D.L. ed. 1989. *Preferred provider organizations: Strategies for sponsors and network providers.* Chicago: American Hospital Publishing, Inc.

Curtiss, F.R. 1990. Managed care: The second generation. *American Journal of Hospital Pharmacy* 47(9): 2047–2052.

Davis, K, G.E., Anderson; D. Rowland, and E.P. Steinberg. 1990. *Health care cost containment.* Baltimore, MD: The Johns Hopkins University Press.

England, B., C., Patterson, and R. Glass (Eds.) 1989. *Quality rehabilitation: Results-oriented patient care.* Chicago: American Hospital Publishing.

Feldstein, P.J. 1988. *Health care economics* 3d ed: New York: John Wiley & Sons.

Fox, P.D., and L. Heinen. 1987. *Determinants of HMO success.* Ann Arbor: Health Administration Press Perspectives.

Gabel, J., and D. Ermann. 1985. Preferred provider organizations: Performance, problems, and promise. *Health Affairs* 4(1): 25–40.

Gannon, J.J. 1985. PPOs: An alternative health care delivery system. *Dimensions in Health Care* 85(1): 1–2.

Gaus, C.R., B.S., Cooper; and C.G. Hirschman. 1977. Contrasts in HMO and fee-for-service performance. *Social Security Bulletin* 40(7): 3–14.

Gold, M. and Hodges, D. 1989. Health Maintenance Organizations in 1988. *Health Affairs* 8(4): 125–138.

Greenberg, I., and M.L. Rodburg. 1971. The role of prepaid group practice in relieving the medical care crisis. *Harvard Law Review* 84: 887–1004.

Group Health Association of America, Inc. HMO Industry Survey 1990. *HMO industry profile*. Washington, DC: Author.

Gruber, L.R., M. Shadler, and C.L. Polich. 1988. From movement to industry: The growth of HMOs. *Health Affairs* 7(3): 197–208.

Harris and Associates. 1984. *A report card on HMOs: 1980–1984*. Menlo Park, CA: The Henry J. Kaiser Family Foundation.

Health Insurance Association of America. 1990. *Source book of health insurance data*. Washington, DC: Health Insurance Association of America.

Held, P.J., and U.E. Reinhardt. 1980. Prepaid medical practice: A summary of findings from a recent survey of group practices in the United States. *The Group Health Journal* 1(2): 4–15.

Higgins C.W., and E.D. Meyers. 1986. Transformation of American health insurance: Implications for the hospital industry. *Health Care Management Review* 11(4): 21–27.

Hodges, D.; K., Camerlo, and M. Gold. 1990. *HMO industry profile: Volume 2, Utilization patterns, 1988*. Washington, DC: Group Health Association of America, Inc.

Houck, J.B., and T.R. Mueller. 1988. Conversion of charitable HMOs to for-profit status. *GHAA Journal* 9(1): 43–56.

Jones, K.R. 1990. Feasibility analysis of preferred provider organizations. *Journal of Nursing Administration* 20(1): 28–33.

Kongstvedt, P.R. 1989. *The managed health care handbook*. Rockville, MD: Aspen Systems.

Langwell, K.M. 1990. Structure and performance of health maintenance organizations: A review. *Health Care Financing Review* 12(1): 71–79.

Lazenby, H.C. and S.W. Letsch. 1990. National health expenditures, 1989. *Health Care Financing Review* 12(2): 1–26.

Levit, K.R., H.C. Lazenby, S.W. Letsch; and C.A. Cowan. 1991. National health care spending, 1989. *Health Affairs* 10(1): 117–130.

Luft, H.S. 1978. How do health maintenance organizations achieve their 'savings'? Rhetoric and evidence. *New England Journal of Medicine* 298(24): 1336–1343.

Luft, H.S. et al. 1980. Health maintenance organizations. In J. Feber, J. Holohan, and T. Marmor (eds.), *National health insurance: Conflicting goals and policy choices*. Washington, DC: The Urban Institute. pp. 129–180.

Luft, H.S., and R.H. Miller. 1988. Patient selection in a competitive health system. *Health Affairs* 7(3): 97–119.

Madison, D.L. and T.R. Konrad. 1988. Large medical group-practice organizations and employed physicians: A relationship in transition. *Milbank Memorial Quarterly* 66(2): 240–282.

Miller, J.L. 1989. New product imperatives and the exclusive provider organization. in D.L. Cobbs, (ed.), *Preferred provider organizations: Strategies for sponsors and network providers*. Chicago: American Hospital Publishing, Inc. pp. 147–162.

Palmer, A.R. 1985. *Economics of participation in preferred provider organizations.* Santa Monica, CA: Rand Corporation.

Pennsylvania Medical Care Foundation 1978. Prepaid health care primer for practicing physicians: Health maintenance organizations and individual practice associations. *Pennsylvania Medicine* 82(9): 10–15.

Richardson, W.C. 1980. Financing health services. In S.J. Williams and P.R. Torrens (eds.), *Introduction to health services.* New York: John Wiley & Sons. pp. 287–322.

Schafer, E.L., C.J., Olson; and M.C. Gocke. 1987. *Evaluating the performance of a prepaid medical group: A management audit manual.* Denver: Center for Research in Ambulatory Health Care Administration, Medical Group Management Association.

Shouldice, R.G., and K.H. Shouldice. 1990. *Medical group practice and health maintenance organizations.* New York: Information Resources Press.

Taylor, H. and M. Kagay. 1986. The HMO report card: A closer look. *Health Affairs* 5(1): 81–89.

Thomas, D.L. 1980. Individual practice association (IPA) model health maintenance organizations (HMOs). *Issues in Health Care* 1(1): 34–36.

Tibbitts, S.J. and A.J. Manzano. 1984. *Preferred provider organizations: An executive's guide.* Chicago: Pluribus Press, Inc.

Wilensky G.R. and L.F. Rossiter. 1986. Patient self-selection in HMOs. *Health Affairs* 5(1): 66–80.

Wolinsky, F.D. 1980. The performance of health maintenance organizations: An analytic review. *Milbank Memorial Quarterly* 58(4): 537–587.

SECTION TWO

THE NURSE'S ROLE

The current health care delivery system and its providers are facing numerous challenges and multiple, complex issues that are the result of the rapid changes occurring in medicine and technology, in societal expectations, in organizational structures, and in resource availability (Ball etal. 1991). Consequently, the intense demands being made on health care organizations and providers, especially nurses, are increasingly complex and volatile. The complexity is a result of the intense focus on balancing quality, productivity, and flexibility in the health care delivery system. Therefore, before discussing specifically the role of the nurse in managed care, a review of the role of the nurse in today's rapidly changing health care delivery system is presented.

Environmental Changes

Changes occurring in the health care delivery system as a result of pressures to contain costs are forcing professionals to change their practice styles and delivery modes. One of the areas experiencing tremendous change is the hospital sector, historically a major employer of nurses. Under current pressures from all sides to use health care resources more efficiently and effectively, patients are admitted to hospitals in a later stage of disease or illness. Today, patients are being cared for as long as possible in a less resource-intensive, noninstitutional health services environment. As a result, the patients who finally are hospitalized are more acutely ill and "their treatment involves a high level of technological care that requires counter-balancing by 'high touch' on the part of nursing staff" (McCloskey and Grace 1990, 166). Also, in response to these environmental pressures for efficiency and effectiveness, patients are being discharged from the hospital sooner, which means they are sicker when they reenter the community.

This hospitalization phenomenon of delayed entry and quicker community reentry increases dramatically the need to coordinate the health care services available outside the hospital setting. Because of the structure and incentives of managed care organizations, there is a strong focus on delaying or avoiding the need for institutional services, with corresponding focus on quality ambulatory care. In this noninstitutional setting, the nurse, as the health professional who focuses on meeting the needs of the client as a person, is increasingly viewed as the individual "to bring coherence to a chaotic and fragmented system of care" (McCloskey and Grace 1990, 166).

To meet these new professional demands, nursing practice must undergo major transitions. Especially now during increasingly limited health care resources, the nurse is key to the necessary processes of efficient resource allocation, coordinated care planning, and essential documentation of outcomes (Mowry and Korpman 1986). In addition, today's nurse is also being asked to justify the costs associated with the provision of quality nursing care (Mills and O'Keefe 1991). It is no longer sufficient for the nurse to document that nursing care impacts positively on patient outcome; the nurse must also document that nursing care is the most cost-effective way of achieving the desired outcome.

Nursing

Throughout time, nursing has been defined by many to reflect the direct interaction with the client. The definition of nursing that reflects this historical orientation, as well as the influence of nursing theory that is part of nursing's evolution is: *Nursing is the diagnosis and treatment of human responses to actual or potential problems.*

"Nursing addresses itself to a wide range of health-related responses observed in sick and well persons. Those responses can be reactions to an actual problem, such as a disease, or they can anticipate a potential health problem. The difference between the response to a health problem and the problem itself is worth noting, as it is here where an intermeshing and complementarity of the distinct foci of the practices of nursing and medicine occur. Human responses to health problems, the phenomena to which the actions of nurses are directed, are often multiple, episodic, or continuous, fluid and varying, and are less discrete or circumscribed than medical diagnostic categories tend to be" (American Nurses Association, 1980, 10).

Nursing Process

Definition

The nursing process provides a coherent, theoretical framework, or model, for appropriate and effective nursing action. A process can be defined as a series of actions that move forward from one point to another on the way to completion of a goal. In a process, there is continuous progress through stages, each stage being dependent on the other and leading to a specific result, outcome, or product. In every process, there is a moving force that controls and systematically directs activities so that the goal is achieved, the defined results obtained. The actions taking place in a process are deliberately and consciously carried out in a logical way. If a process is without a goal or there are no deliberate efforts to achieve it, the process has neither meaning or substance and will sooner or later break down (Keane 1986, 9). The goal that the nursing process is directed at achieving is the alleviation, minimization, or prevention of health problems at both the individual and population level. The nursing process makes nursing practice focused, comprehensive, rational, methodical, effective, and consistent, which ultimately should improve the quality of patient care (Derdiarian 1991, 2).

Structure

In general, the process of nursing is viewed (Keane 1986; Mowry and Korpman 1986; McCloskey and Grace 1990; Scherer 1986) as consisting of four fundamental parts: assessment and diagnosis, planning, implementation and documentation, and evaluation. The nurse uses these four basic components to develop and implement a plan of patient care designed to meet the specific health needs of an individual client. "The various elements of the nursing process enable the nurse to identify the needs of the individual patient and his family, to establish priorities and goals, to carry out the plan of care, and to develop alternative plans of action in response to changing needs and to evaluate the results of nursing intervention" (Scherer 1986, 346). As this explanation implies, the nurse is not only concerned with an individual patient, but also with the patient's family. The nurse also tends to be concerned in designing a care plan with the social environment as well as the medical conditions of the individual in mind. Not all nurses perform the same scope of practice in this process; an individual nurse's scope will depend on his or her education, previous experience, personal skills, specialization, and the policies and structure of the organization in which the nurse is employed (Tranbarger 1991).

The first stage of the nursing process is *assessment and diagnosis*. During this stage, the nurse assembles and analyzes subjective (patient perceived) and objective (observable, verifiable) information from a variety of sources for the purpose of identifying and understanding the client's problems and their underlying causes. The nurse uses this information to formulate a nursing diagnosis, which describes the patient's problems (Keane 1986). The nursing diagnosis is different from the medical diagnosis in that it goes beyond the identification of a disease and focuses on the contributing personal, family, and social aspects of the illness.

The second stage of the nursing process is *planning* the patient's nursing care plan or intervention strategy, which outlines the nursing actions to be undertaken to meet the total needs of the patient based on the information obtained during the assessment and diagnosis stage. During this stage, the behavioral objectives or expected patient outcomes are realistically formulated from information obtained during the first stage. The planning function continues throughout the nursing process as plans change to adapt to the patient's unique needs (Mowry and Korpman 1986).

Implementation and documentation is the third stage of the nursing process. During implementation, the actions outlined in the nursing care plan are carried out. Accurate and timely documentation of what actions are to be carried out, who is responsible for each action, and how the patient is expected to respond to each action (and then how the patient actually responded) is essential to maximizing the effectiveness of the care. Information on the response to specific actions must be communicated to all members of the health care team if knowledgeable and appropriate decisions are to be made (McCloskey and Grace 1990). Thus, documentation of activities and reactions is essential in the provision and continuity of high-quality care.

During the final stage, *evaluation*, the outcomes achieved during the implementation stage are compared with the goals formulated during the planning stage. If the actual outcomes do not correspond to the goals established, then this evaluation process enables the goals to be reassessed and redefined or for alternative plans to be formulated and implemented. Evaluation also provides an essential contribution to the continuity and quality of care provided and to the measurement of quality (Scherer 1986).

Pressures for Change

Today's turbulent health care environment is placing substantial pressure on nursing to demonstrate and document the effect that nursing care has on patient outcomes and on the economic efficiency and price competitiveness of services provided. It is imperative that nurses be able to document the unique elements of nursing and to demonstrate that the benefits achieved with those elements exceed the costs incurred in providing nursing care. In addition, for those elements of nursing that are not unique to the profession, nurses must be able to demonstrate that they can render the services more cost effectively than other providers.

The nursing process outlined above provides an excellent framework for meeting this challenge. As demographic and societal changes continue to occur—(changes in the demographic profile of the population; increases in chronic illnesses; increased emphasis on noninstitutional provision of health care services; changes in health care organizational structures and financing mechanisms; changes in societal expectations of the health care system)—increasing demands will be placed on nursing and on nurses to address these changes effectively and efficiently.

Managed Care

The emergence of managed care organizations provides opportunities, challenges, and potential threats for nursing (LaBar and McKibbin 1986). The goal of these organizations—to manage the utilization of appropriate health services by individual members—is consistent with the basic philosophy of nursing, which focuses on the total needs of the individual, not just on a disease. There is also goal congruence between nursing and the managed care organization to maintain the health of the individual in order to minimize the need for expensive health care services. Within this structure of managed care, however, there is also a need for strong professional advocacy on the part of nurses to ensure that the organization does not underserve the needs of the individual member as it strives to control costs. In meeting the needs of the organization and of the members, the nurse also plays an important role in managing resources.

Role in Managed Care

The following sections demonstrate the wide scope of functions and activities nurses perform in managed care organizations. Although the functions and activities discussed in these sections are not exhaustive, they do illustrate many of the opportunities, challenges, and threats for nursing offered by this form of health care delivery system. Also, although these functions and activities are presented as discrete units, they often overlap or are interdependent. As a result, the role of the nurse will usually encompass more than one of these functions and activities simultaneously.

Primary Care Provider

Primary care refers to a type of health care services and a way of delivering those services. It is the care the client receives at the first point of contact with the health care system that leads to a decision of what must be done to help resolve the presenting health problem. It also is continuous and comprehensive care, including all the services necessary for health promotion, prevention of disease and disability, health maintenance, and in some cases, rehabilitation. Primary health care includes identification, management, and/or referral of health problems, as well as promotion of health-maintaining behavior and prevention of illness. It also is holistic care, which takes into account the needs and the strengths of the whole person. Since primary health care involves the delivery of health care from entry into the system and is also continuous and comprehensive, it necessitates collaboration among many health professionals (Council of Primary Health Care Nurse Practitioners 1985, 1).

Primary health care is a fundamental service of managed care organizations as they attempt to minimize the need for more specialized, resource-intensive services. In addition, nurses have an important role in the delivery of primary health care in managed care organizations. As these organizations focus on providing necessary services in the most cost-efficient manner, they attempt to utilize the least costly combination of resources to achieve the desired goal. As a result, in collaboration with physicians and other health professionals, the nurse is involved in assessing and managing a wide range of acute and chronic illnesses in managed care organizations.

In their concentrated efforts to provide comprehensive, cost-effective, quality health care, managed care organizations are often more creative in their use of various health professionals. This flexibility in meeting the needs of their members enables them to maximize the capabilities of all health professionals in the delivery of services (Gluck 1980). The central concentration of resources and personnel of the more structured managed care organizations (that is, staff, group, and network model HMOs) is especially conducive to the delegation of responsibility to the most cost-efficient, medically appropriate provider of health services. The central concentration of resources increases the ease of using internal consultations and collaborative endeavors in meeting the needs of their members.

Since a primary focus of managed care is on helping people to know when, where, and how to receive health services in efficient and cost-effective ways, there is a major role for nurses in the delivery of primary care. In managed care organizations, as in traditional settings, nurses are recognized as experts at being able to manage the care provided to clients across clinical settings (Holt 1990). In addition, nurses provide a variety of health promotion, prevention, and maintenance services to a wide range of patients. The potential delegation of responsibility to nurses for the provision and coordination of primary care services is tremendous. In general, nurses in managed care organizations perform health assessments, monitor chronic illnesses, provide direct patient care for acute problems, and provide education to patients regarding a wide range of issues (Davis 1990).

Study after study has been conducted (Fagin 1982; Record et.al. 1981; Sox 1979; Weiner, Steinwachs, and Williamson 1986) demonstrating that utilizing nurses, especially nurse practitioners, in the provision of primary care is a cost-effective way of maintaining and even improving the quality of care provided to members of managed care organizations. These studies also have shown that, in general, patients have been very satisfied with the services received from these providers, and the members indicate that they are receptive to the increased use of these nonphysician providers in the delivery of primary care.

As medical technology evolves and financial incentives change, increased emphasis is placed on providing services to patients outside the resource-intensive institutional setting. Consequently, current patients seen in an ambulatory setting or in the home require nurses to have the knowledge and skills necessary to manage seriously ill individuals. Many of these noninstitutionalized patients require high-technology interventions and sophisticated technical treatments, changing the traditional clinical, counseling, and coordinating roles of the nurse. Today's nurse must also be capable of counseling and teaching patients and their families about these complex techniques, since these individuals are being forced to assume an increased amount of responsibility for actually administering treatment (Salmon and Vanderbush 1990). Nurses are increasingly assuming this role as they provide primary care to members of the managed care organization.

The provision of primary care services requires collaborative efforts from a team of diverse professionals, not just the nursing staff. To be successful, the collaborative team approach must meet the needs (real and perceived) and expectations of the plan members. In addition, the professionals involved must also be satisfied with the care provided and with their role in its provision. There must be open communication among all participants so that everyone is clear about what is being asked of them in the arrangement and what the expected outcomes are. Unless expectations are met, there is potential for conflicts to arise among the professionals, causing dissatisfaction that may spill over into the patient domain (Gluck 1980). Provider dissatisfaction can have a perceived, if not actual, adverse impact on the quality of patient care.

"Managed care has long recognized the talents of nurse practitioners as cost-effective care givers, especially for maintenance of chronic care, and will continue to seek qualified individuals to deliver these services. Because business and industry are now encouraging the use of managed care, it follows that nurses will be increasingly recognized as cost-effective providers of services" (Davis 1990, 355). As pressures continue to control the costs of health care services, nurses will increasingly be viewed as critical professionals in the delivery of cost-effective health care services.

A large ambulatory care center operated by a multistate HMO illustrates how a team of certified nurse midwives and obstetricians/gynecologists reduced the length of hospital stay after delivery, decreased the use of epidural anesthesia, and increased utilization of the HMO's free-standing birth center, all cost-reducing activities (Stewart 1988). Instead of fostering competition among these types of providers, the team approach emphasizes how these different professionals supplement and complement each other's practice. This leads to improved provider and patient satisfaction as physicians care for and counsel patients with high-risk OB/GYN problems and nurse midwives care for and counsel healthy mothers throughout pregnancy, offering clinical, social, and emotional support and providing routine gynecological services. In addition, the members of the plan "appreciate the time that CNMs [certified nurse midwives] take to answer their questions, teach new concepts, and provide health care. At the same time, they appreciate the security of the physician back-up for complicated OB/GYN problems" (Stewart 1988, 8). In this managed care organization, the team participants are comfortable with their collaborative roles because expectations are clearly defined concerning each of their roles in the process and the individual and overall outcomes to be achieved.

Another facet of primary care offered by nurses in managed care organizations involves home health services. In today's world under managed care systems, the nurse is truly accountable for planning and executing the care of patients at home. The total number of visits for a spell of illness is limited by the third party payor, but the skilled, professional nurse has the opportunity to devise a plan of treatment that offers patients and families the support needed for independence at home. Under a "managed care system," as it is defined today, patients need not receive less nursing care, but better organized care (Daniels 1988, 18–19). In a managed care plan, the primary care nurse is responsible for ensuring that each member visit to the plan results in maximum effectiveness in patient outcome and satisfaction and that the most cost-effective alternative for monitoring patient progress and compliance is utilized.

Another area where nurses have been used extensively in managed care organizations is in the provision of pediatric care. In managed care organizations, as in other practice settings, the pediatric nurse has had to adapt to the results achieved with extraordinary medical technology innovations. As advances in medical technologies enable more and more infants and children with major medical problems to survive for extended periods of time, attention must be focused on meeting their needs by providing "comprehensive, cost-effective health care in an environment that maximizes individual capabilities and minimizes the effects of the disabilities" (Eck and Ryan, 1990, 212). Pediatric nurses will increasingly play an important role in managed care organizations in determining how the health care services provided to children are managed, distributed, and provided.

As technologies evolved enabling pediatric services to be provided outside an institution, nurses in managed care plans increasingly assumed the responsibility for assessing the capabilities of families to care for the patient and for teaching the necessary skills for caring for the patient in the home. In addition, "nurses, as direct-care providers, must take a much more assertive role in the case-by-case decisions regarding the applications of technology. Through relationships with the family and colleagueship with physicians, nursing is in a unique position to influence directly the application of the human side to the technology. Nursing can help the family and other health team members to examine critically the options for care as they relate to the potential outcomes" (Eck and Ryan 1990, 215). Just because technology is available does not mean that it is appropriate in every circumstance.

As these examples demonstrate, nurses play a critical role in the delivery of primary care services in managed care organizations. Time after time it has been shown that using nurses in the provision of direct patient care enhances the quality of care and increases the level of recipient satisfaction. (See, for example, Council of Primary Nurse Practitioners 1985; Daniels 1988; Davis 1990; Holt 1990; Stewart 1988). The appropriate utilization of nurses results in effective, efficient health care services.

Case Manager

Managed health care organizations rely on case management as one strategy for controlling costs, reducing inappropriate utilization of services, and improving quality of care. HMOs and PPOs engage the services of case managers to manage the care of and costs to members with catastrophic illnesses and injuries; high-user, high-risk, or high-volume members; members with chronic and disabling conditions; and members whose cases are projected to cost $25,000 to $50,000 a year. Case managers are also used when cases are identified as having a high likelihood of exceeding any annual or lifetime plan benefit limits that might exist (Like 1988). Managed care organizations, especially HMOs, have much stronger capabilities to perform this function because of the link between the system's delivery and financing components.

For case management to strike a balance between the costs and the quality of health care delivered for complex and difficult cases requires the involvement of multiple health care disciplines and a case manager who works collaboratively with the patient's primary care physicians, the patient, family members, and other providers both within and outside the plan. The goal of case management is to achieve the desired outcome for the individual member while using the appropriate amount, type, and sequencing of resources (Fondiller 1991).

How case management functions in a managed care organization will depend on the type of organization involved (HMO or PPO) and who bears the financial risk for the case. In PPOs, which generally are not financial risk-bearing organizations, case management services can be provided by the PPO itself, by a contracting utilization review company, by the payer/carrier, or by another independent agency on contract with the PPO. In some PPOs, case management is offered as a supplemental service and provided on a fee-for-service basis for the PPO, the carrier, or the employer, depending on who pays the bills.

In HMOs, which by their very nature bear the financial risk of providing services, case management services generally are provided by the medical services department, which is also responsible for providing utilization review and quality assurance services. In most HMOs, case management services are provided at the sole discretion of the medical director and nurses are generally charged specifically with carrying out this task (Coleman 1990).

Although case management services are offered by some PPOs, this is not as common as it is in HMOs. As discussed previously, the financial risk of such costly and complex cases is usually not borne by the provider-sponsored PPOs (a separate insurance company usually retains financial risk). The provider-sponsored organizational form currently accounts for more than one-half of the PPOs in existence (HIAA 1990).

Case management as a professional practice is still in its infancy. Although some (Fondiller 1991; Knollmeuller 1989) have suggested that case management has been around since the turn of this century in the form of public health nursing, the concept is now being redefined; there are more definitions being put forward today by different organizations, providers, and health care professionals than ever before (Cline 1990; Faherty 1990; Knollmeuller 1989; Scully and Nichols 1990). Case management has been defined generically by Weil and Karls (1985) as: ''a set of logical steps and a process of interaction within a service network which assures that a client receives needed services in a supportive, effective, efficient, and cost-effective manner'' (p. 4).

While there is a great deal of variation in how case management functions in managed care plans, the problem-solving methodology used is generic and is derived from the nursing process. Generally, case management includes the following steps or functions (Shipske 1982):

- intake
- assessment
- development of a care plan
- referral and follow up
- case coordination
- implementation of the plan of care
- ongoing assessment
- plan of termination
- case recording/reporting
- supervision of workers on the case
- quality assurance for the case.

The case manager in a managed care organization tracks the patient through the various units of the system, thus enhancing continuity of care. The patient care plans developed during this process identify a "critical pathway" of key events that must occur in order to achieve the desired outcome in a timely manner. The nurse case manager oversees these critical paths and facilitates interventions to ensure that the patient progresses through the desired events appropriately and satisfactorily (Fondiller 1991).

Quality of care is also improved through the continuity of care provided with case management. Especially in the ambulatory setting of managed care organizations, case management addresses the long-term needs of the enrolled members, not just their current interaction with the system. This is particularly true in the management of patients with chronic medical problems. Continuity of services is also improved since a single individual is responsible for ensuring that the prescribed plan is followed or adapted as necessary by integrating the individual parts of the system (del Togno-Armanasco, Olivas, and Harter 1989). Through coordination activities performed by the case manager, fragmentation and duplication of services are avoided.

When nurses perform the activities of case management, they are fulfilling the functions of what the American Nurses Association (1988) has described as nursing case management: "a health care delivery process whose goals are to provide quality health care, decrease fragmentation, enhance the client's quality of life, and contain costs" (p. 3). To achieve these goals, case managers are called on to do more than just simply coordinate the needed services of a patient. In fact, the role of a case manager has evolved into a pivotal one of problem solving and managing both the cost and quality of needed health care services.

Part of the duties of the nurse case manager is to educate the patient. The nurse explains the concept of case management, the progression of care that can be expected, and the anticipated outcomes. The nurse case manager is also available to answer any questions the patient may have. In addition, the case manager performs a supportive role during patients' interaction with the health care system: Their adherence to the treatment regimens can be improved simply because they are being monitored and their concerns attended to during entire care process (McKenzie, Torkelson, and Holt 1989).

The actual role of a case manager is dictated by the patient's specific needs. For example, if a patient has a post-acute problem, such as a stroke, the case manager may only need to coordinate the rehabilitation services of several health care professionals (home health nurses, occupational therapists, speech therapists, durable medical equipment specialists) for a short period of time.

Another patient may have more severe problems, such as a spinal cord or head injury, and therefore require extensive intervention and more supervision. In this instance, the case manager has to be concerned with a more complex plan of care, along with more medical, nursing, and financial management. This patient's condition may not improve quickly and may even worsen over time. In this situation, the case manager will have to explore several cost-saving opportunities and negotiate services and prices for many different health care professionals and suppliers over an extended period of time and across the entire care continuum. Often, severe conditions become more complicated because of benefit limitations, exclusions, and life-time cost limits, all of which must be factored into an optimal solution for the member and everyone else associated with the case (McKenzie, Torkelson, and Holt 1989).

In the management of chronic illnesses such as chronic obstructive pulmonary disease, diabetes, multiple sclerosis, arthritis, or cancer and of acute episodes of these illnesses, the case manager's role is to coordinate and provide needed services to maintain these patients outside of the inpatient institutional setting for as long as possible, but not necessarily to rehabilitate them. The case manager's role with high-risk infants and high-risk pregnancies is somewhat different. In these instances, the goal is to keep the presenting condition or problem stabilized so the patient can go home or stay home and not require expensive inpatient services.

As these cases illustrate, case managers are called on to do more than simply coordinate needed services of one or more health care providers. In most catastrophic and large-claim cases, the case manager must coordinate the services of health care professionals from multiple provider organizations, as well as negotiate payment terms and conditions, the duration of services, and possible changes in the member's benefit coverage (del Togno-Armanasco, Olivas, and Harter 1989). For example, additional services, including some that would not ordinarily be covered by the member's medical benefit plan, may be recommended in order to keep the member at home or in a lower-cost treatment facility or program. This extension of benefit coverage may be the only possible way to keep costs below an annual or lifetime limit imposed by the managed care plan's coverage.

This coordination activity inevitably requires artful negotiations with the insurer/HMO, primary care provider, patient, family members, and a host of other providers. Clearly, the role of the case manager varies from case to case. Generally, however, the case manager helps all of the affected parties stay within the HMO's provider network, optimizes utilization of the benefits of the plan, and ensures observance of any plan cost limits, while at the same time balancing quality of care and member advocacy to meet the expectations both of the member and of the managed care organization.

The types of cases and the number of parties responsible for the costs of the services influence the roles the case manager assumes and the degree of involvement of other interested parties. Following is a list of the major types of cases that are most commonly referred to a case manager because of complexity, high use, or high cost.

- AIDS
- amputations
- connective tissue diseases
- congenital deformities
- end-stage cancer
- head injuries
- multiple fractures
- multiple sclerosis
- multiple trauma/spinal cord injuries
- neonatal high-risk infants
- organ transplants
- paralytic disorders
- renal disease
- severe burns
- terminal illness
- ventilator dependency.

In managed care organizations, these cases usually are referred to the case manager by either the utilization review nurses, the primary care physician, the medical director, or the claims department. In those managed care organizations that require hospital preadmission authorization or referral certification and authorization, these cases are usually identified quickly and referred to the case manager for early intervention and follow-up. Of course, early discovery and referral to case managers saves the most dollars and permits the case manager, along with the member's primary care physician, to better manage the care and costs of the situation. Early intervention by case managers allows more controls to be put into place to prevent the medical and cost situation from worsening, to achieve efficient and prudent use of the plan's provider network and benefits, and to stretch the managed care plan's benefit dollar.

The clinical experience and problem-solving and business skills needed to balance both caring and business aspects of difficult and complex situations varies with the degree of autonomy given to the case manager and the number of roles he or she is called on to assume. In most referral situations, the case manager acts as a consultant and is given the authority to search for the one best clinical and business solution and to recommend to the managed care plan what should be done to care for members within the plan's benefits coverage (Shipske 1982). In addition, the case manager is expected to report on the options that may exist outside the plan should utilization of out-of-plan services be the only way to balance care, costs, and quality.

The clinical and business skills required to do the job are also greatly influenced by the goals of the organization employing or engaging the services of the case manager, as well as by the amount of financial liability it has for the case at hand (Like 1988). When a nurse is employed by an HMO, he or she will from time to time have to coordinate activities with several other people within the organization. For example, the case manager may have to work simultaneously with several in-plan and out-of-plan health care professionals and agencies, including the following (Cline 1990):

- the member's primary care physician
- the medical director, if the case is extremely complex
- the patient's spouse or other family member
- a social worker or hospital discharge planner
- home health nurses and therapists
- community and voluntary health agencies.

The case management process is not unique to managed care organizations, but the economic importance of such a strategy to managed care intensifies its utilization in these organizations (Coleman 1990). The roles that the case manager must assume in managed care plans are not unique, but occur in other practice settings and include the following (Coleman and Hagen 1991):

Facilitator: The case manager facilitates the entire case management process and gets all of the affected parties working towards mutually agreed upon goals.

Liaison: The case manager is a formal communication link between the patient, his or her primary care physician, all in-plan and out-of-plan providers, the medical director, and plan management.

Coordinator/Gatekeeper: The case manager helps the patient get through the health care delivery maze by arranging, regulating, and coordinating the needed health care services at all the necessary points of service.

Broker: The case manager brokers provider services that are needed to meet the patient's needs and to stay within any coverage or budget cost limits imposed by the member's medical plan or HMO.

Educator: The case manager educates the member, family, and providers about case management, the health care delivery system, community health resources, and benefit coverage so that informed decisions can be made by the affected parties.

Negotiator: The case manager helps negotiate the plan of care, services, and payment arrangements with providers and, sometimes, benefit coverage changes with the HMO.

Monitor/Reporter: The case manager acts as a feedback loop for the HMO, reporting on the status of the member and situations that affect patient safety, care quality, patient outcome and that will increase costs and the HMO's liability.

Patient Advocate: The case manager acts as the patient's advocate, providing information and support and, at times, obtaining additional benefits, extended benefits, or services that might not ordinarily be covered simply because of their cost but that benefit the member, family, primary care physician, and HMO.

In performing these various roles, the nurse case manager balances costs with quality and works to apply strict interpretations of ''medically necessary'' for the HMO. At the same time, the nurse case manager looks at the needs of patients and their families as they cope with extremely difficult and costly situations.

Another function that case managers undertake in managed care plans is the standardization of the appropriate use of services and treatments. The focus of this standardization feature is on improving service volume management, reducing variation of resources used in providing care (del Togno- Armanasco, Olivas, and Harter 1989). Standardization usually results in the formation of specific time-sequenced care plans (often called critical path plans) that identify the type and timing of care in order to comply with typical treatment modalities for a specific type of patient. These standards do not replace individualized care, but target deviations from the standards so that the resources used can either be justified or modified. Standardization can also improve quality of care as variations are quickly observed during monitoring and the problems can be resolved or remedial actions taken immediately (Fondiller 1991). This promptness can significantly enhance the quality of care provided, as well as its cost effectiveness.

The nurse case manager's job is not easy. He or she must always be current with new advances in medical treatment or diagnostic technologies, state-of-the-art home medical equipment, new drug regimes, and the standard of medical practice in the community (Daniels 1988). The nurse case manager must also be innovative and creative in terms of identifying all feasible solutions and selecting the one solution that appears to satisfy the most parties. The case manager must satisfy many different people yet remain objective, not become codependent on the patient, and somehow satisfy both the patient and the HMO when catastrophes strike.

Figure 3 illustrates how the patient and the case manager become the center of attention of everyone who is affected by the problem or condition and the many forces that define the feasible solutions and that affect the selection of the optimal clinical and business solution for all of the parties involved. It is evident from this illustration that a successful case manager must be able to shift gears and combine clinical nursing knowledge with sound business practices and apply good economic decision making in the search for the optimal solution.

While searching for the right clinical and financial outcome, the case manager may have to conduct treatment research and perform several benefit-cost analyses. When this is necessary, the case manager will have to determine the financial impact of a case for different and sometimes innovative care plan approaches and for different time periods (Coleman 1990).

For example, a case manager may have to determine and negotiate the cost of continuing care in the hospital and compare it against the cost of providing care in either a skilled nursing facility or in the patient's home. For high-risk or ventilator-dependent patients, this might require comparing the cost of a continued stay in an intensive care unit for several weeks to the cost of providing high-tech nursing around the clock at home.

Figure 3: **Forces Affecting Solutions**

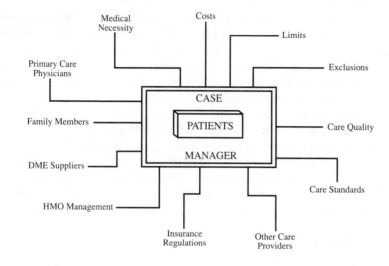

Case managers must have good business acumen to negotiate fixed and favorable prices with in-plan network providers and other community providers in trying to extend a patient's benefit and stretch the HMO's benefit dollars or reduce its financial liability.

Case managers typically are called on to solve the most difficult problems of the managed care organization. Some problems are the result of high costs; some are caused by communication problems between patient and physicians; still others are the result of repeated inappropriate use of medical resources by patients or plan physicians.

Participation in case management programs can, however, lead to greater professional and personal satisfaction for nurses. By overseeing and coordinating a complete episode of care, the nurse gains greater control over an important nursing aspect—caring for the patient. According to McKenzie, Torkelson, and Holt (1989), nurses have cited ownership, recognition, and increased involvement with management as important benefits of participating in a case management program. Collaborative interactions with physicians are also enhanced with the multidisciplinary approach as physicians feel more confident that the prescribed treatment plan designed to meet all the patient's needs will be carried out efficiently and effectively. Through case management, the chief benefits of managed care have been identified as shortening the length of stay of patients in hospitals, reducing the adverse outcomes experienced by patients, strengthening collaborative practices, and

improving resource allocation by determining appropriate tests and procedures (Fondiller 1991).

Nurses are in a unique position to function as case managers.
"Nurses are the generalists; they are the detail people, and they excel in
managing care. They are at the juncture of cost and quality, and they
know the human implications of trade-offs such as early discharge,
patient education in groups, or the use of new technology. Most important are two underlying elements: 1) nurses use the formal nursing
process, which is directly analogous to the process of case management;
and 2) nurses are committed to the welfare of the institution and, with
support, are willing to assume more authority in the smooth, integrated
management of patient care" (Zander 1990, p. 201). The case management process addresses the issues of resource allocation, effectiveness of
care, cost containment, and accountability—all important elements in an
efficient and effective managed care organization.

Patient Advocate

A major role of the nurse is patient advocacy. This role is especially
important in managed care organizations where the nurse often
assumes responsibility for ensuring that the member's long-term needs
are met. An advocate has been defined as "one who works with or on
behalf of a person or system to bring about a positive difference in the
system's state or the individual's condition of health" (Brill and Kilts
1986, p. 77). When acting as a patient's advocate, the nurse may be
providing direct care to the patient or acting on behalf of the patient in
interactions with others in the managed care system.

The basic functions performed by the nurse advocate are to inform
and support. "Briefly, the role of the advocate is to inform the client and
then to support him in whatever decision he makes" (Kohnke 1982, p.
2). The nurse advocate helps the patient explore the options available
and then supports the patient's decision once the patient has made an
informed choice about which option to pursue. In helping the patient
carry out the choice made, the nurse often must act as an interpreter and
intervenor within the managed care plan to enable the patient to implement the desired choice in the most effective and efficient way. In this
role, the nurse may perform such activities as identifying and referring
the patient to appropriate resources and services; manipulating schedules to best meet the patient's needs, desires, and requirements; and
acting as a spokesperson for the patient with other personnel and components of the managed care organization and system (Brill and Kilts
1986).

In assuming the role of patient advocate, the nurse must be cognizant of the demands of such an undertaking. The necessary knowledge

to perform this role is tremendous. The nurse must be informed about available and appropriate treatments, medications, and procedures so that such information can be conveyed to the patient; have the skills to present the information in such a way that the patient understands the ramifications of each alternative; and be able to convey the necessary information in a non-judgmental fashion so that personal biases or concerns do not unduly persuade the patient to select a particular option (Kohnke 1980).

In addition, finding the time to perform the advocacy role is extremely demanding. The nurse must find the time to become fully informed about the options available for the patient, both professionally and organizationally, and then to inform the patient about all of the options available and each of their ramifications. The nurse must also allow time for the patient to ask questions to enhance an understanding of the information conveyed. The goal is to have an informed patient, which implies understanding, not just a patient with information (Kohnke 1982).

The nurse advocate must also realize that others within the managed care plan may simultaneously be acting as the patient's advocate. Consequently, the plans, goals, and interventions of everyone involved must be coordinated. To be effective, the nurse advocate must use judgment, creativity, and problem-solving skills to negotiate a successful solution for everyone involved. To achieve the best results, the nurse must act through collaboration rather than confrontation. As an advocate for the individual, "the nurse informs others in the health care system of the actions, confers with others to find means of carrying out the individual's informed choices, checks information and clarification, and respects others' opinions, viewpoints, and expertise in the option process" (Brill and Kilts 1986, p. 78).

The following discussion illustrates the patient advocacy role of the nurse in negotiating a successful solution to an analgesic regimen that was not working for a particular postoperative patient. According to Walker and Wong (1991), the management of pain begins with four "rights" —the right drug, the right dose, the right time, and the right route. If there is inappropriate deviation in any one of these elements, the pain management regimen will not be successful.

When the patient complained of pain, the nurse checked to see if the patient's prescription allowed some flexibility in terms of dose or time. The nurse found that such flexibility did exist and, working within the existing structure, increased the dose and decreased the time between doses in an effort to manage the patient's pain. When neither of these two modifications alleviated the problem, the nurse then proceeded to determine what drug therapy alternatives were available for this particular patient and to document carefully and thoroughly an analysis of the possibilities. After all possible alternatives were identified and analyzed, a specific drug, route, time, and dose likely to manage the pain of this patient, and the reasons for their selection, were well documented. This information was then presented to the physician in a nonconfrontational way, resulting in the recommended change in the analgesic regimen (Walker and Wong 1991). In this instance, the informed, well-organized nurse was able to persuade the physician to change the analgesic regimen to enhance the care provided to the patient.

As a patient advocate, however, once an individual patient has made an informed choice among possible alternatives, the nurse must provide active support for that individual's decision, even if that decision is in conflict with the personal preference of the nurse in terms of treatment modality or alternative. The nurse advocate must remember that his or her approval of the patient's decisions is not required; what is required is acceptance of the patient's right (and responsibility) to make decisions (Van Kempen 1979).

At times, the role of the nurse advocate for an individual member may be in conflict with the goals of the managed care organization and the benefit constraints of the plan. These conflicts are not unique to managed health care, and their resolution requires collaboration, not confrontation. It must be remembered that the organization is also interested in providing quality care and in keeping members satisfied with the services provided. The managed care organization sees the nurse advocate as a very important mechanism for increasing quality and improving public credibility (Wiseman 1990). However, balancing the needs of the individual and the needs of the organization requires careful negotiations.

Patient Educator

As the major medical problems addressed by the health care system shift from acute illness to chronic conditions, the focus of the system must also change. Instead of providing cures or preventive measures, medical intervention is increasingly directed at helping individuals manage their own chronic diseases. As patients assume more responsibility for maintaining their own health, the role of the educator in including the patient as a team member in the health care process will grow.

Patient education has been defined as: ''the act or process of providing patients with knowledge, skill, competence, or desirable qualities of behavior'' (Harper 1976, p. 2). The goals of patient education are to promote health, maintain or improve current health status, and encourage involvement in self-help endeavors (Keane 1986). In general, patient education is a constellation of interventions that encourage and promote self-modifications, value clarifications, and sensory preparations.

Since many of the chronic medical problems encountered today are affected by lifestyle and personal choice, a major concern of health education is to address these risk factors. Another major concern is patient noncompliance with a treatment plan, which often results in relapse and additional utilization of the health care system—an expense the managed care organization wishes to avoid for itself and for its members. In terms of reasons identified for noncompliance, "one of the major causative factors was a lack of understanding of what was being done and why it was important" (Rowland and Rowland 1985, p. 496). Consequently, a successful patient education program focuses on helping the individual understand the risk factors involved and assume responsibility for certain aspects of the health care plan.

The nurse has an important role in this education process since he or she often spends substantially more time with the patient than do other professionals on the health care team and in the managed care system. This increased contact results from managed care organizations supporting the patient-education role of the nurse, therefore allowing the nurse more time to fulfill this function. Since the nurse has the most extensive contact with the plan member, he or she can plan and implement both formal and informal programs. In addition, the nurse educator can adapt the education process to meet the member's specific needs and to recognize the most effective ways of educating the patient (Redman 1980). The nurse usually has contact with family members and can include them in the education process to help carry out the instructions concerning the intervention strategies.

A primary feature of any managed care organization is the education of its members as it strives to reduce its members' needs for expensive health care services. Therefore, managed care organizations place emphasis on "communication of information, recommendations of behavior change, personal reassurance and support, and coordination of diagnostic and therapeutic interventions" (Davis 1989, p. 54). Although patient education is the responsibility of everyone within the managed care organization, it is often the nurse who assumes responsibility for coordinating the education process to send a consistent message.

In helping patients improve their health or cope with their limitations, nurses perform two roles: "first, as a facilitator, to facilitate the learning/ performing of self-care measures; and second, as a consultant, to help patients in the decision-making process where their health is concerned (O'Connor 1990, p. 145). The role of the nurse, therefore, is to ensure that appropriate opportunities are available within the managed care system for the patient to learn the necessary information to achieve the desired level of functioning. If the organization supports only the education of individuals with serious levels of a chronic illness, for example, then the newly diagnosed patient may not receive sufficient information to delay progression of the disease or to avoid complications. Insufficient information leads to long-term increased costs and decreased quality for the patient and for the organization. To avoid these results, the managed care plans allow nurses the time and opportunity to provide comprehensive patient education.

As managed care organizations attempt to improve the efficiency and effectiveness of the services they provide, patient education programs have been shown (Boyd etal. 1991; Davis 1989; O'Connor 1990; Redman 1980; Rowland and Rowland 1985) to be major contributors to the process. "Patient education facilitates shortened hospital stays, reduces post-operative complications and pain, and helps restore activities of daily living. Aside from the satisfaction nurses experience when patients respond to their teaching efforts, such efforts increase patients' sense of control through mutual participation in health care" (Boyd etal. 1991, p. 89). This sense of control is reinforced when health education clarifies the dynamics and processes of health care. When patient education efforts are coordinated so that materials are repeated and reinforced consistently, the results are beneficial to everyone involved.

Patient education does not always have to be a formal and structured process. As nurses interact with patients throughout the managed care process, the education they provide can be integrated through role modeling and direct contract. Nurses can capitalize on educational opportunities spontaneously as they occur.

The following examples illustrate how nurses can use the informal process to educate patients. "For example, while using a glucometer to measure the blood sugar of a patient recently diagnosed with diabetes, a nurse could recite the steps aloud as initial preparation for the patient to develop self-care abilities. In another instance, a nurse could briefly explain to an edematous patient the rationale for fluid restriction, and then place the intake and output record at the bedside" (Boyd etal. 1991, p. 89). These are just two examples of how a nurse can be alert and take advantage of education opportunities that arise during their interactions with patients. These spontaneous and indirect forms of education are a critical aspect of the nursing process and, furthermore, they enhance the welfare of the patient, the nurse, and the organization. Effective health education programs can reduce the number of broken appointments, improve patient compliance with medical regimens, decrease morbidity and mortality among members, and improve acceptability of care (Arnold 1981).

In addition to educating patients, the nurse educator has a crucial role in educating (both formally and informally) other members of the staff to enhance their teaching and communication skills. The nurse educator also serves as a valuable resource for formal educational program development and as a resource for effective techniques in the teaching-learning process (O'Connor 1990). The effectiveness of patient education programs can be greatly enhanced when all personnel in contact with the patient reinforces the desired message in a consistent manner.

Triage

An important function in managed care organizations is ensuring that members receive timely access to the appropriate level of health care services. A strategy often employed to direct patients through the system is to use a triage nurse to handle telephone calls and on-site visits from members who present with sudden problems, either real or perceived. Triage is defined as "a process by which a patient is assessed upon arrival to determine the urgency of the problem and to designate appropriate health care resources to care for the identified problem" (Bailey, Hallam, and Hurst 1987, p. 65).

The provision of clinical and/or counseling services through medical telephone calls plays a significant role in the American health care system. Overall, approximately 20 percent of all physician-patient encounters occur in this form; the relative importance of this service delivery mode varies by specialty. "Among primary care specialties, telephone calls account for 19.4% of all patient encounters in family/ general practice, 24.6% in general internal medicine, 28.5% in pediatrics, and 19.6% in obstetrics/gynecology" (Radecki, Neville, and Girard 1989, p. 817). These authors also reported that almost half of the medical telephone contacts are managed solely by telephone and the other half are a prelude to an office visit; in pediatrics, over 60 percent of such calls are managed solely by telephone. Using a triage nurse in a managed care organization to screen these medical telephone calls can have a substantial impact on efficiency in the plan. Decreasing the demands on physicians' time will require fewer physicians (a very expensive resource) to be employed by the plan.

In a managed care organization, the triage nurse listens to the member describe the problem and symptoms, and, if necessary, reviewing the member's medical record on file in the central system. He or she decides what course of action—immediate intervention, intervention within 24 hours, routine appointment, or no intervention—is most appropriate and then advises the member accordingly. This mechanism for directed access to safe and appropriate health care services achieves more efficient and effective utilization of the health care delivery system and hence improves the use of resources (Winder 1990).

Triage nurses provide short-term, episodic intervention to plan members and facilitate access to the appropriate service point in the health care system. The role of the triage nurse in the managed care plan is "to negotiate a satisfactory resolution with a caller whose expectations may be unrealistic" (Scott and Packard 1990, p.3). The triage nurse, therefore, uses different diagnostic skills than those needed when providing direct patient care. In triage, instead of diagnosing a disease, the nurse is diagnosing the presenting symptoms in terms of appropriate access and negotiating with the member to help them reach a mutually satisfactory decision. "The registered nurse is primarily responsible for assessing the urgency and severity of the problem and for providing an appropriate disposition based on that assessment" (Group Health Cooperative of Puget Sound 1984, p. xiv).

One of the most important characteristics of a good triage nurse is effective communication skills. Since the majority of the triage nurse's contacts with members are by telephone, it is crucial that the triage nurse establish an atmosphere of openness, receptiveness, reassurance, and mutual trust (Scott and Packard 1990). It is paramount that members feel that the triage nurse is trying to help them achieve effective and efficient utilization of appropriate services that is mutually satisfactory, and not simply trying to deny them access to care in order to contain costs for the managed care organization. By communicating effectively with the members in resolving the problem, greater compliance with the decisions reached can also be achieved.

Protocols are often utilized by nurses in managed care organizations, as in other settings, to help explore the problem and gather the necessary information to arrive at an appropriate assessment. The nurse should not use this tool as a substitute for eliciting comprehensive information about the various members' symptoms and their emotional context. But protocols can be used to ensure that nothing important is omitted in the assessment process. "Protocols provide triage guidelines for callers with specific problems and associated symptoms" (Scott and Packard 1990, p. 41).

Protocols are written strategies for determining of the urgency of the problem and aiding in the disposition of the patient. In most settings, protocols have been developed to help the nurse handle the following adult and pediatric health problems (Group Health Cooperative of Puget Sound 1984):

- The problem occurs frequently in outpatient care and is often amenable to home treatment without the intervention of a physician.
- The problem is urgent or emergent and requires skilled nursing assessment and intervention to improve outcome.

- The problem has been diagnosed previously by a physician and the patient is seeking additional information.
- The problem requires referral for medical information.

The use of written protocols in reaching a decision can often improve the decision quality, especially since protocols establish a systematic thought process. The written strategies, however, do not replace the skills and expertise of the triage nurse.

Once the problem has been identified and the triage category established, the next step is to communicate the solution to the member in a mutually satisfactory way. As the triage nurse interacts with the member of the managed care plan, the possible options within the triage category identified should be presented. The nurse should then help the member reach a mutually satisfactory decision and encourage compliance. It is crucial that the member be satisfied with the solution reached and, again, not feel that necessary health care services are being denied solely for the financial benefit of the managed care organization.

Quality

Concerns about the quality of care delivered are not unique to the participants in managed care organizations; however, many of the inherent features of managed care organizations—discounts, utilization management, restricted professional autonomy, risk contracts, capitation, restricted access, limitations on provider choice at point of service—make them targets for increased scrutiny and accusations of decreased quality (Boland 1991). As a result, both internal and external efforts are focused on ensuring that quality is not compromised by the organization's emphasis on managing care and controlling costs, and that accurate and appropriate information about quality of care is conveyed to the public. A major problem encountered in trying to ensure quality, however, is the lack of a commonly accepted definition and quantifiable measure of quality. Without a common definition, documentation and measurement is difficult.

According to Boland (1991), the issue of quality should be assessed along six dimensions:

Control: inspection of the production process to detect possible defects and problems.

Assessment: identification of outliers from formulated selected clinical indicators and establishment of intensive review procedures for the outliers.

Assurance: identification of good clinical standards and evaluation of providers' performance relative to standards.

Improvement: translation of quality into on-the-job expectations for all individual work functions and installation of greater inter-dependence through team-building within the organization.

Treatment outcomes: measurement of the effect of medical intervention on patient status in terms of clinical indicators, functional status, access, appropriateness, and satisfaction.

Treatment analysis: determination of whether poor outcomes were due to patient, physician (and other care givers), or system problems.

As these factors illustrate, quality is multidimensional and its definition, measurement, and evaluation is complex. There is not a single uniformly accepted measure that can be used to indicate that quality care has been provided to a specific individual or to the population in general. "But the most important fact is that performance data relating to quality is the very substance of what managed care is supposed to be" (Boland 1991, p. 11). The goal of managed care organizations is to provide quality care in a cost-effective way. When quality of care is being evaluated, consumers' perceptions regarding service quality are just as important as the clinical features of quality—perception is reality.

With the increasing emphasis on quality, a variety of control programs have been developed and introduced. "The term quality control is a management term that denotes a management process designed to evaluate and monitor the quality of a product. Originally used in industry, quality control has now been applied to health care and hospitals. It refers to a set of functionally related activities that evaluate, monitor, or regulate the quality of services rendered to the consumer. Both management and clinical processes are included. The quality control activities are commonly referred to as quality assurance" (Sliefert 1990, p. 234). The fundamental components of any quality control program are: 1) to set standards; 2) to compare actual performance to the standards established; 3) to introduce a plan of action to change deviant behavior; and 4) to provide feedback regarding the actions undertaken.

In setting the standards of practice in the health care field, three basic audits are used: structure, process, and outcome. "The structure audit is concerned with the setting in which care is given. Structure audits focus on physical facilities, equipment, the personnel giving the care, and the organization of the institution. This involves looking at rules and policies governing the professional work and medical records and is based on the assumption that, given reasonable (according to current perceptions) standards of facilities and organization, good medical care is likely to prevail" (Hartman 1976, p.2). However, there is no documentation of a direct relationship between excellence in structure and excellence in quality of care.

"The second type of audit is the process audit. Under this approach, the auditor focuses on what happens and the order in which events occur. Information for process audits is collected either by direct observation or by record review, which may be done retrospectively or concurrently" (Hartman 1976, p.3). The process audit is task oriented and difficulties are encountered in evaluating the quality of the activities performed instead of just documenting the performance of the activity.

"The third type of audit has only fairly recently been developed. This is the outcome audit, which looks at the status of the patient as a result of the care provided. This type is most frequently done retrospectively and asks: What effect did the care given have on altering the health status of the patient? A problem of outcome audit is the difficulty in defining 'outcome'" (Hartman 1976, p.4).

Regardless of the actual process used in quality assurance programs, the goal is to hold health care professionals and organizations accountable for the quality of the care they provide. To be effective, the professionals providing the services must know the standards and criteria to which they will be held accountable in the internal and external review processes. In this way, the professionals can use the information provided to improve the quality of the services they provide.

Nursing has a significant role to play in each phase of the quality improvement process. Since nurses are heavily involved in many different aspects of the delivery of health care services in managed care organizations, they also are involved in identifying the problems or topics to be evaluated in the quality improvement process. Nurses in managed care organizations are involved in formulating the measures that will be used to reflect quality care as quality relates to a particular practice issue; this is especially true in the identification and measurement of quality nursing care. These measures of quality of care reflect standards of care, or the levels of care expected (Araujo and Jurkovic 1984). The involvement of nurses in this process, thus ensuring that professional assessment and judgment will be incorporated in the design and execution of the process thus ensuring excellence in the health care services provided in the managed care plan.

In the pursuit of quality, an important structural component involves the professional qualifications of the people providing services. The selection of providers and the ongoing evaluation of their performance are essential inputs into quality care; but these inputs alone are not sufficient to guarantee quality. An appropriate mix of number and type of providers supports the ability of the managed care organization to render quality health care (Ebers and Smith 1989). Highly trained nurses are used effectively to evaluate the credentials of personnel within the managed care organization and to establish the performance standards for assessing, monitoring, and improving ongoing evaluations of these personnel.

While the following description of the credentialing process refers specifically to physicians, the concepts and criteria are appropriate for other health professionals in the organization as well. The physician credentialing plan should include evidence of education, training, experience, licensure, board certification, and existing inpatient clinical privileges. Satisfactory recommendations of professional performance, clinical skills, ethical character and ability to work with others are essential components of the plan. Malpractice experience and insurance coverage should also be considered. Compliance with the plan's bylaws, rules, and regulations; participation in required continuing medical education programs; patterns of adverse clinical outcomes; evidence of satisfactory performance and clinical judgment are additional factors to take into account (Ebers and Smith 1989, p. 94). As this discussion indicates, a comprehensive credentialing plan is a critical foundation for quality care.

Medical care evaluation is another component of quality assurance in managed care organizations, as in other settings. The first step in a comprehensive medical care evaluation is to establish a detailed set of criteria for establishing the standard of care relative to a particular subject. Next, "medical records of patients with appropriate diagnoses are then reviewed against the agreed upon criteria and assessments are made. The reviewer uses branched chain criteria (e.g., if A was found, was B done?)—in short, a sort of 20 questions" (Kongstvedt 1989, p. 115). Deviations from these established criteria for standards of care can be viewed as initial indicators of low-quality care and, if necessary, appropriate remedial actions can be taken by the managed care plan to improve the care provided.

Another component of quality assurance in managed care plans is peer review. "Peer review is the act of physicians reviewing each other's medical records and passing judgment on them, or at least provoking useful clinical discussions based on those records. Because it is so potentially threatening to physicians, peer review is always in danger of deteriorating into a mutual toleration society" (Kongstvedt 1989, p. 116). While the previous statement refers only to physicians, peer review activities should be undertaken by all other professionals with direct responsibility for the outcome and management of cases. To be effective, peer reviews must generate discussion among the participants about the appropriate management of the case. The peer review process also serves as a backup mechanism for problems identified in the other components of quality assurance. A formal peer review process is essential in imposing sanctions for poor-quality care delivered within the managed care organization.

In addition, the managed care organization must have an effective, formal process for addressing member complaints. Although the members may not possess the knowledge to evaluate technical quality, their perceptions of service quality form the basis for their satisfaction and future participation in the plan. "The plan should also perform studies that look at the criteria many members use to judge the quality of care themselves (i.e., appointment availability, waiting times, cleanliness of offices, telephone responsiveness, and on-call availability)" (Kongstvedt 1989, p. 117). The information gathered from these routine studies can then be used to enhance the practices of the providers in the system. Consumer expectations should be linked to provider performance. Nurses in managed care organizations are, therefore, critical components of this quality assurance process.

As should be apparent from these quality assurance techniques, quality does not just happen; it must be planned. "In both the service and manufacturing sectors, one of the keys to quality is the culture of the organization and how well it supports the efforts of various groups of employees to work together" (Ersoz and Forney 1991, p. 417). In this interrelated quality assurance process, Crosby (1980) has identified four absolute definitions of quality:

1. Quality has to be defined as conformance to requirements, not as goodness.
2. The system for causing quality is prevention, not appraisal.
3. The performance standard must be zero defects, not "that's close enough."
4. The measurement of quality is the price of nonconformance, not indexes (p. 58).

"The price of nonconformance in health care organizations relates both to issues of risk management and prevention of lawsuits, and to the lower cost of getting it right the first time" (Ersoz and Forney 1991, p. 418). The goals should be to avoid defects rather than to correct them. Quality assurance programs, therefore, should be directed at eliminating defects or barriers to quality so that the system is designed to maximize the quality of care. Nurses provide crucial input into the identification of the points in the managed care system where improvements can be made to improve the organization's ability to deliver quality health care services.

In adopting a quality control program, the focus should be on assessing accuracy, completeness, correctness, cost, and timeliness of the activities performed "The terms 'cost of poor quality' or 'price of nonconformance' grew out of initial industrial efforts to quantify the economic benefits of initiating and sustaining total quality management initiatives. Identifying the costs associated with the failure to meet customer requirements, with duplication of efforts, and with re-work is an important element of clinical continuous quality improvement" (Kralovec, Huttner, and Dixon 1991, p. 3).

The measurement of quality in the managed care organization should be related directly to monitoring conformance to the goal of system restructuring to improve performance in order to meet all customer requirements (Kralovec, Huttner, and Dixon 1991).

The focus of quality assurance is on increasing the probability of achieving the desired outcomes in patient care services. "Quality assurance is a combination of interrelated activities whose primary focus is to assess and evaluate patient care. ... Quality assurance is best described as a process-oriented, clinical function performed by a wide range of medical practitioners" (Schuler 1991, p.54). In managed care organizations, nurses play a vital role in performing quality assurance activities.

Resource Management

The organizational and financial structures of managed care organizations make it imperative that they provide quality care in the most effective and cost-efficient way possible. Therefore, a primary responsibility of administration in managed care organizations is to seek ways of improving the organization's performance. To achieve effective and efficient delivery of care, a systematic and ongoing effort to plan, monitor, and control resource utilization and acquisition must be undertaken. This effort is crucial if the organization is to balance the goals of mission, quality, and profitability. To ensure that the resources of the organization are controlled and utilized appropriately, some type of a formal utilization management process is necessary.

Utilization management includes both authorization systems and utilization review mechanisms. "Utilization management is a mechanism for managing health care costs by assessing the appropriateness of care and influencing decisions about its provision to ensure the least costly but most effective treatment. Thus, while primarily focused on reducing costs, utilization management also affects quality of care" (Tischler 1990, p. 1099). The foundation of the utilization management process involves judgments of the clinical appropriateness of the care provided; therefore, the process has implications for quality of care as well as cost containment.

"Utilization management is an adjudicative process that applies a 'clinical' means test to justify admission and establish the appropriate level of care, to evaluate the medical necessity of specific services and procedures, to ascertain that services are provided in a manner consistent with accepted standards of care, and to ensure the timely implementation of the treatment plan" (Tischler 1990, p. 1100). In general, the determinations are made by comparing the current situation to preestablished criteria. Obviously, a crucial component of the process is the validity of the criteria applied to the clinical situation. An effective utilization management program enables the organization to allocate its limited resources to maximize benefits to members and to the organization.

One of the definitive elements of an effective utilization management program is some form of an authorization system that defines services, procedures, and activities that require authorization as well as those that do not. "The tighter the authorization system, the greater the plan's ability to manage utilization. An authorization system per se will not automatically control utilization, although one could expect some sentinel effect. It is the management behind the system that will determine its ultimate effectiveness" (Kongstvedt 1989, p. 143).

An important component of the managed care plan's authorization system is determination of who within the organization has the ability to authorize services and to what extent. The more tightly controlled the authorization system, the more services requiring authorization.

In many managed care organizations, the primary care providers are delegated the responsibility for authorizing all nonprimary care services, except for special conditions reserved for the medical director. To be most effective in controlling utilization, the primary care provider must also act as case coordinator or "gatekeeper" and authorize any additional services requested by the referral provider.

"In any type of managed care plan, there may be services that will require specific authorization from the plan's medical director. This is usually the case for very expensive procedures such as transplants, and for controversial procedures that may be considered experimental or of limited value except in particular circumstances. This is even more necessary when the plan has negotiated a special arrangement for high-cost services. The authorization system not only serves to review the medical necessity of the service, but ensures that the care will be delivered at an institution that has contracted with the plan" (Kongstvedt 1989, p. 144). In defining the services requiring the authorization of the medical director, it is necessary to balance the controls established with the time and cost commitments of such approval activities.

For control purposes, the authorization system may be classified into three major categories: prospective, concurrent, and retrospective. By categorizing the types of authorization required, monitoring will enable the plan to determine if, in fact, the system is operating in the desired way.

Prospective authorization is issued before the service is rendered and is also called precertification. The most common type of service requiring prospective authorization is an elective service, especially one performed on an inpatient basis. "The review considers the necessity of the admission, the appropriateness of types of admission, and the completeness of preadmission evaluations. In determining the necessity of admission, the review certifies that the activities of the proposed admission must be done in the hospital and cannot reasonably be done in an ambulatory setting because of patient safety or logistics. ... The determination of the appropriateness of the type of admission focuses on the use of the hospital inpatient facilities immediately preceding or following a diagnostic procedure or surgical treatment. ... The determination that all appropriate preadmission workup is completed confirms that diagnostic testing and consultations can be done before proceeding with the proposed hospital treatment. Additionally, confirmation of preadmission workup establishes that the results of such testing are available and have been reviewed. Finally, it confirms that all arrangements for using the operating room or other hospital services have been completed" (Cowan 1984, p. 170–171).

In addition to inpatient services, prospective authorization can be used for many types of ambulatory care services and procedures. The goal of prospective authorization is to decrease the inappropriate use of resource-intensive services and shift the site and type of service to the most cost-efficient, medically effective location. Nurses, with their philosophy of holistic health care and clinical education, are often utilized by managed care organizations in performing the prospective authorization activities.

A second general category of authorizations is *concurrent*, and these authorizations are generated at the time the service is rendered. These authorizations usually occur when the service is considered urgent and the primary care provider makes a referral and contacts the plan authorizing the service at the same time. "Concurrent authorizations allow for timely data gathering and the potential for affecting the outcome, but do not allow the plan medical managers to intervene in the initial decision to render services. This may result in care being inappropriately delivered or delivered in a setting that is not cost effective, but also may result in the plan's being able to alter the course of care in a more cost-effective direction even though care has already commenced" (Kongstvedt 1989, p. 145). In conducting concurrent authorization reviews, the nurse reviewer focuses on determining the most effective way to manage the course of care from that point on.

Retrospective authorizations occur after the service has been rendered. If prospective and concurrent authorizations are properly obtained, retrospective authorizations should occur only in cases of emergency or an urgent problem that occurs outside the plan's service area. Even in such cases, there should be preestablished provisions for systematic notification to the plan in a timely manner, and the utilization of the services should then be reviewed for medical necessity and appropriateness. The automatic review of all such cases should not be interpreted to mean automatic approval; the nurse reviewer should closely monitor the cases by member and by provider to identify potential patterns of misuse of the system. Once identified, appropriate corrective actions can be taken.

The data provided by the authorization system should enable the nurse reviewer to link claims data to authorized services within the plan. The data and reports generated should be used to identify noncompliant providers and providers submitting requests in an untimely manner. These data are critical for active medical management by the plan.

A second major tool of an effective utilization management program is the utilization review process. Although utilization review is essential for cost control, it also monitors the quality of care provided by the plan. If the utilization review process is extensive and comprehensive, then efficient, quality practice will be stimulated. Within the utilization review system, there are two major categories of review: concurrent and retrospective. While some authors include prospective review, this mechanism really refers to an authorization technique rather than a utilization review technique.

Concurrent review involves analyzing the use of resources, the timeliness with which treatment is provided, and the adequacy and timeliness of discharge planning. Concurrent review in the hospital applies to all patients, that is, those admitted on an emergency or urgent basis as well as those admitted electively. It involves certifying the necessity of the admission and assigning a length of stay to each patient based on reason for admission, diagnosis, and severity of illness. Concurrent review also involves a daily determination that necessary tests are ordered and performed in a timely manner and that unnecessary tests are not done. It also requires a daily determination that proper and appropriate treatment is initiated without unnecessary delay (Cowan 1984, p. 172).

Although this discussion applies to hospitalization, the same types of concurrent review can be applied to the services provided on an ambulatory basis. The nurse uses concurrent review to analyze critically the member's progress toward the desired outcome. Concurrent review provides opportunities for the team of professionals to make changes in the member's ongoing treatment plan, which can not only reduce the resources being utilized but also improve the quality of care provided.

Utilization review is very appropriate in an ambulatory setting, but it is harder to accomplish there than in an inpatient setting given the nature of ambulatory services. Since the outcome in ambulatory care is hard to define and to affect, it is difficult to establish quantifiable review criteria. The people obtaining services in an ambulatory setting often have either self-limiting diseases or chronic conditions, where treatment is often palliative (Benson and Townes 1990). Thus, measuring the results of the care is complex in ambulatory care settings. However, since this is the setting in which a majority of managed care members seek care, it is imperative that a successful utilization review process be developed. In establishing the criteria to be applied in evaluating the appropriateness and necessity of ambulatory services, incorporating the knowledge and experiences of nurses is crucial. Managed care organizations often allow nurses to spend more time than other professionals with members, so their insights into the treatment process are very important.

For the hospital patient, *discharge planning* is a critical component of concurrent review. It involves evaluating the patient, family, and home situation to establish the types of services and arrangements that will be needed when resource-intensive hospital care is no longer appropriate. Discharge planning should be started at the time of admission if not before so that adequate arrangements can be made.

Discharge planning substantially increases continuity of care. "An effective discharge planning program provides the mechanism for targeting groups of patients with specific needs who can be cared for in alternative settings" (O'Hare and Terry 1988, p. 15). Not only does discharge planning improve quality of care by ensuring that the appropriate types and sites of care are rendered, it is also essential to the financial health of the organization. "Nursing's involvement recognizes the quicker-and-sicker nature of patients leaving the hospital today. Nurses must be part of discharge planning in order to assess the medical and nursing needs of patients, to discuss and alert physicians about the various levels of care and sites available, and to coordinate the detailed and technical services needed by these patients" (O'Hare and Terry 1988, p. 39).

The discharge planner associated with a managed care organization can coordinate the services for members so that services are provided effectively and efficiently. When nurses perform the duties of discharge planning, they make use of the nursing process—assessing, planning, implementing, and evaluating—to develop a patient care plan that will meet the needs of the patient in the most cost effective manner. These nurses also ensure that the treatment plans are individualized and clinically appropriate, and that they adhere to the clinical standards of the profession and the organization (Meisenheimer 1985).

The following example illustrates how discharge planning can modify practice patterns and encourage the appropriate utilization of the least resource-intensive services. It also illustrates that granting exceptions to the plan's contract may be beneficial to both the member and the organization.

A fourteen-year-old covered dependent was hospital-confined in an acute care facility for treatment of major depression, alcohol/drug abuse, and a conduct disorder. A case manager began case activity with the assistance of a local psychiatric nurse consultant. The possibility of discharge planning was discussed with the treating psychiatrist and although the case manager had made no discharge plan before intervention, the nurse consultant was able to assist the psychiatrist in setting discharge goals.

Case management included extensive involvement with the dependent's family, the treating psychiatrist, and the psychiatric nurse consultant. With the nurse consultant's input, an outpatient program was developed that provided a structured and controlled environment. Benefits for the outpatient program were provided outside the policy contract. This outpatient program is an alternative to inpatient care and, with the close monitoring and additional benefit coverage, the dependent was maintained on an outpatient basis.

In this case, discharge planning enabled the member to be treated in a less restrictive and less resource-intensive setting. As long as such a setting is medically appropriate and the outcome achieved is comparable, the cost savings to the plan should become part of the decision making process.

"Retrospective review is the traditional form of utilization review in which clinical decision making and the use of services are evaluated after services have been provided" (Cowan 1984, p. 172). *Retrospective review* can be applied not only to the appropriateness of specific services, but the data collected can be used to analyze the frequency of services utilized by specific providers and members, and providers' use of ancillary and consultative services, medications, and emergency room services (Cowan 1984). These practice profiles can then be used as educational tools in modifying provider behavior to achieve the desired results.

When conducting retrospective review, it is important to remember that the goal is to improve the cost efficiency and effectiveness of the services provided and to improve the utilization of resources in providing health care services; the attitude should not be one of "gotcha." Through providing comparative information on how resources are utilized by other providers within the system, provider behavior can be modified. The system should not be viewed as punitive, but rather as supportive. Of course, if certain providers do not modify their behavior once deviations are pointed out, then corrective actions will need to be taken.

Many managed care organizations employ a utilization review (UR) nurse to assist in meeting the requirements of utilization management. "The UR nurse makes use of the nursing process (assessing, planning, implementing, and evaluating) to develop a patient plan of treatment as well as review plans for each service providing care... The UR nurse ensures that the care is individualized and clinically appropriate, and adheres to clinical and regulatory standards" (Stone and Krebs 1990, p. 15). The utilization review nurse can also act as consultant to other service providers to establish treatment plans that best meet the needs of the members within the constraints of the organization. As managed care organizations attempt to face the challenge of providing quality, appropriate, cost-effective care to their members, the role of the utilization review nurse is to provide creative, functional strategies for meeting this challenge.

Risk Management

A function that is tied closely to quality improvement and utilization management is risk management. While the focus of quality improvement is on increasing the probability of achieving a desired outcome, the focus of risk management is on decreasing the probability of incurring an adverse one.

Risk management is a process through which risk to the organization "and all who are associated with or served by it are evaluated and controlled in order to reduce or prevent future loss. A comprehensive program includes primarily control of professional liability but also incorporates other elements, such as environmental safety, security measures, and infection control, to name a few. While risk management involves the evaluation, treatment, and financing of present loss, the key is in controlling the possibility for loss. Therefore, successful risk management includes identifying and analyzing potential risk and developing subsequent preventive measures" (Culp, Goemaere, and Miller 1985, p. 170).

Although the overt orientation of risk management is administrative and focused on the reduction of the organization's exposure to risk, patient welfare is its foundation. When the organization is able to control risk, quality of care is enhanced. This quality enhancement maximizes the welfare of the patient, and, ultimately, of the organization (Culp, Goemaere, and Miller 1985).

All risk management processes perform four basic steps in their efforts to protect against events that jeopardize the operations of the organization: identification, analysis, evaluation, and treatment (Schuler 1991). Step 1, *identification* of sources of risk for the organization, should be a proactive activity rather than waiting for something to occur and then trying to fix it. Because nurses have direct access to and responsibility for patient care, they are in an excellent position to identify potential risk factors and to determine what situations that do occur may be detrimental to the patient. Risk and uncertainty can never be eliminated, but their early identification can minimize their occurrence and their negative impacts. According to O'Hare and Terry (1988), at least the following items should be identified with risk management screens:

- unclear intake/referral/feedback criteria
- untimely or delayed discharge planning activity
- improper utilization or malfunction of equipment
- potential for inadequate or unsafe vendor services
- improperly trained staff
- use of lower-level staff to give high-technology care
- inadequate insurance coverage for independent contractors
- inadequate communication with referring physician (p. 143).

Once potential risk factors have been identified, the second step, *analysis*, should be performed to increase understanding of the sources of risk. The analysis identifies not only individual events, but patterns and frequencies of events and possible system design defects contributing to their occurrence. During the analysis step, traits of patients susceptible to high-risk events can be developed and environmental elements contributing to high-risk events can be categorized. Nurses can contribute substantially to this analysis because of their background and involvement in patient care.

Following analysis, *evaluation* is conducted to formulate alternative approaches to reducing the identified risks. During evaluation, suggestions and observations are solicited from a wide variety of sources. Nurses are major contributors during this step because of their involvement in multiple areas and functions throughout the organization. The suggestions and observations are utilized to formulate intervention strategies.

The fourth step, *treatment*, involves implementation of corrective intervention strategies to reduce the risk factors. These treatments may result in changes in policies, protocols, practice patterns, or system design. The goal is to modify current operations in order to reduce, if not eliminate, unsafe conditions and thereby prevent injury and subsequent loss. The outcome of a successful risk management program is improvement in patient care. As Duran (1980) noted, "The way the nurse relates to the patient may make the difference between a lawsuit and one that never happens." Risk management activities, therefore, do not have to be formal, elaborate affairs but they do need to involve everyone in the organization.

Many organizations establish a position titled "nursing risk manager". This individual assumes many responsibilities, including (Culp, Goemaere, and Miller 1985):

- identifying the frequency of preventable events
- reducing the severity of preventable events
- minimizing losses and damages
- developing risk management education programs
- providing safety program guidelines
- initiating appropriate, efficient, timely actions to correct problems
- documenting and reporting incidents
- providing internal communications
- gathering information to prevent recurrence
- providing a vehicle for suggestions to improve quality
- identifying adverse patterns regarding incidents
- alerting management to system design problems
- developing management reports and recommendations
- analyzing elements contributing to incidents.

The nursing risk manager does not perform these functions in isolation. To be most effective, risk management must be coordinated with other quality assurance and utilization review functions and its implementation must be a collaborative effort.

Benefits Interpreter

By their nature, managed health care organizations limit access to health care services; therefore, these organizations need a mechanism to explain their authorization and control functions to the members and to handle any complaints and grievances that arise. The purpose of these mechanisms is to enhance the level of satisfaction between the members and the organization.

As the managed health care industry evolves, boundaries blur, and plans add new features and options to their established benefits package, it is crucial that the schedule of benefits available under each option be clearly defined and well documented. As new members enroll and existing members select different options, the specific schedule of benefits available to them must be clearly explained. In addition, as members utilize the system, it is also important that providers be aware of the restrictions of the plan so they can rationally discuss the options available to the member. Most members are willing to accept the restrictions if they have been carefully and fully explained (Daniels 1988).

To enhance member satisfaction and increase compliance with plan restrictions, a comprehensive outreach program is extremely useful. "An outreach program is one that proactively contacts new members and discusses the way the plan works. By reaching out and letting members know how the authorization system works, how to obtain services, what the benefits are, and so forth, the plan can prevent confusion. This also gives the member a chance to ask questions about the plan, especially when those questions don't come up until the member has heard about the plan from the outreach personnel" (Kongstvedt 1989, p. 167). Prior understanding of the restrictions and conditions of participation will lead to increased satisfaction with service quality, higher retention, and decreases in complaints and grievances.

An area requiring special attention when interpreting benefits is the issue of medical necessity, which is the criteria normally used to determine if an intervention is covered by the plan. Theoretically, medical necessity reflects the biotechnical criteria determining if a specific intervention is appropriate given the patient conditions and symptoms. It is important to understand, however, that while the term "medical necessity" appears to be based in scientific objectivity, in reality it contains many value judgments and assumptions about how society should function. Medical necessity is not a simple, objective concept. Consequently, there are substantial opportunities for legitimate conflicts to occur among organizations, clinicians, and plan members in interpreting the medical necessity of an intervention (Sabins, Forrow, and Daniels 1991).

In attempting to define medical necessity, many organizations and practitioners go beyond the biotechnical criteria in prescribing or authorizing tests, procedures, and services. For example, although an intervention may not be medically necessary based on biotechnical criteria, it may be viewed as humanly necessary in the developmental process of forming a positive collaborative provider-patient relationship; or, it may be viewed as pragmatically necessary if providing the intervention would require less time, energy, and cost than not providing the intervention; or it may be viewed as personally necessary as defensive medicine against possible malpractice actions (Sabins, Forrow, and Daniels 1991). Each of these definitions of "necessary" raises valid points; therefore, in interpreting the benefits in respect to medical necessity, the individual's unique situation and specific set of circumstances must be carefully considered. In supplying the interpretation, caution must also be exercised that the decision does not set a precedent for a particular class of patients within the plan.

Another area in which interpretation of medical necessity is required is in determination of appropriateness of intervention given the patient's condition and symptoms. The goals of this appropriateness review are to reduce costs and improve quality of care by eliminating the risks, pain, and expense of medically unnecessary procedures. In performing the role of appropriateness reviewer in determining medical necessity, the nurse must assemble clinical data about the patient and then systematically compare those data to predetermined medical indicators, protocols, and standards of care. If there are questions regarding the appropriateness of the proposed intervention, then the case should be referred to a specially trained advisor for additional review and the final decision should involve the provider, the reviewer, and the advisor (Findlay 1989). This process should enable the managed care plan to avoid providing high-risk or inappropriate care to its members. As a result, quality of care should be improved and costs reduced.

Another function of benefits interpretation is to decide when exceptions to the plan's coverage, limitations, and exclusions should be authorized. In deciding if a patient's conditions or circumstances warrant exception consideration, it is critical that the effectiveness and efficiency of the proposed strategy be well documented. The following example illustrates the appropriate use of extracontractual benefits to maximize the welfare of the member and the plan.

An individual was in the final stages of AIDS and was hospitalized. At this point, case management was activated. The claimant's physician had requested authorization to keep the patient hospitalized until his death even though the claimant and the family wished to have the patient discharged home for his final days. The claimant's health policy covered home health care, but limited the care to forty visits per calendar year.

A case management nurse began working with the attending physician, claimant, and family members. All parties agreed that the patient would benefit from going home as long as appropriate home health care was provided. The claimant's employer was consulted regarding the dollar savings anticipated in considering home health care versus continued hospitalization, and the employer agreed to provide extracontractual benefits in order to cover the claimant's home health care needs beyond the forty-visit limitation. The case manager coordinated the extracontractual agreement as well as the management of the home health care agency chosen to provide the nursing care.

The claimant was discharged from the hospital with home health care provided twelve hours per day and supplemental help provided by the family. The patient was able to remain at home until death and the family sent a warm letter of appreciation after his passing.

In this case, the patient's preferences were achieved and the plan was able to reduce costs by authorizing these extra benefits. Since daily hospitalization costs are usually about five times the cost of comprehensive daily home health care, the savings to the plan could be significant. As long as home health care can appropriately meet the patient's needs, then such an exception to plan limitations should be evaluated.

Provider Liaison

The role of the provider liaison is to furnish information to and interact with other health professionals regarding patient-related and administrative issues. This function is crucial in managed care organizations where a variety of health professionals provide services concomitantly to an individual in an effort to achieve the plan's goal of providing efficient, effective, high-quality health services at an affordable cost. As these different health care providers interact, the provider liaison ensures that all participants understand each other's functions and roles. Without this clearly defined understanding, strained relations and confusion are likely to result from role conflicts and turf struggles (Germain 1984).

The organizational structure of managed care necessitates collaboration, cooperation, and coordination among a wide mix of health professionals. Each of these health professionals brings to the organization and to service delivery a specific base of knowledge and competency. A crucial aspect of the liaison function is to ensure that these individual skills are integrated into a cohesive, comprehensive set of services for the members (Schlesinger 1985). Nurses are almost uniquely qualified to perform this integrative role given their clinical training and their holistic approach to patient care. These skills are utilized to prevent duplication, avoid diffusion of professional responsibility, and reduce the chance of miscommunication among the various members of the staff.

Another important aspect of the liaison function is to improve understanding among the various health professionals of the contributions each discipline makes to the overall goal of appropriate member services. For the managed care organization to function most efficiently and effectively, there must be a climate of openness among the professionals. To achieve this openness, health professionals must understand the values, philosophy, skills, and expertise of other participating disciplines and all disciplines must adopt a common "language" when collaborating and cooperating in the provision of health care services to members (Germain 1984). The provider liaison must stimulate, nurture, negotiate, and promote this understanding and openness.

Nurses' Satisfaction

A number of studies (Bunsey et.al. 1991; Carmel et.al. 1988; Geiger and David 1988; Gillies, Franklin and Child 1990; Langenfield 1988; McConnell 1982; Smith 1980; Smith 1981; Stillwaggon 1989) have been designed and conducted to evaluate the level of job satisfaction and quality of working life nurses experience. Several of these studies have attempted to determine what factors are associated (positively and negatively) with the level of job satisfaction and the consequences of dissatisfaction.

In general, the factors contributing to job satisfaction or job dissatisfaction can be classified as physical, social, and emotional (Albrecht 1979).

"Physical factors are those aspects of an individual's environment that cause physical distress or anxiety about possible consequences, including noise, air pollution, radiation, dangerous machinery, physical injury, and serious illness. Social factors involve those aspects having to do with the individual's interactions with other people as a part of living and working in an organization. The organization can be either the home or the work setting and includes family members, peers, head nurse, supervisor, patients or clients, physicians, and committees to which one reports. Albrecht defines emotional factors as 'those abstractly conceived aspects of the individual's relationship to the environment that lead to anxiety, frustration, apprehension, anger, or other stress-derived emotions.' Deadlines, fear of success or failure, success itself, lack of control, ego risk (that is the fear of loss of status or self-esteem), expectation of disapproval from significant others, and extreme accountability for high-task risks are included in this category" (McConnell 1982, p. 111).

All of these factors are interactive and additive as contributors to the level of job satisfaction nurses experience.

Although many of these factors may be outside the direct control of organizations, some can be influenced by the way the organization is structured and administered. Since managed care organizations are under pressures to provide their services cost effectively, these organizations should be especially interested in reducing the results of job dissatisfaction—turnover, absenteeism, impaired employees, errors, member dissatisfaction, increased recruitment and orientation expenses, increased supervision of new recruits. In organizations where individuals must interact with and be dependent on others, the frustrations, anger, anxiety, exhaustion, irritability, nonproductivity, and isolationism resulting from job dissatisfaction will exponentially affect other individuals in the organization (Friel and Tehan 1982). Therefore, administration, which creates the work environment, should develop strategies to minimize the negative impacts of that environment on employees and improve the quality of working life.

The quality of working life has been defined as "the degree to which members of a work organization are able to satisfy important personal needs through their experiences in the organization" (Hackman and Suttle 1977, p. 4). In a health care organization, the results of poor-quality working life can be disastrous to the quality of services provided and, ultimately, to the continued survival of the organization. Since nurses perform such critical roles in managed care organizations, their inability to render high-quality care may jeopardize the welfare of the entire organization. Consequently, in evaluating managed care, it is crucial to evaluate the quality of the nurses' working life.

In evaluating the quality of working life in managed care organizations, three behavioral dimensions should be measured: 1) job satisfaction; 2) organizational commitment; and 3) job tension (Porter et al. 1974). These behavioral dimensions are highly interrelated. Job tensions negatively effect job satisfaction and loyalty to the organization. Although job satisfaction does not guarantee commitment and continued employment, job dissatisfaction does increase the probability that the employee will leave the organization, an expensive event. Lower job tension and higher job satisfaction and organization commitment do improve performance outcomes, resource effectiveness, and quality of care (Smith 1980).

In order for managed care organizations to achieve their goals of high-quality, cost-effective health care, the individuals working in these organizations must be satisfied with their work environment. Otherwise, the potentially superior organizational and financial qualities of managed care organizations will not be realized and their performance will be suboptimal (Smith 1980). There must be a balance between meeting personal and organizational goals for success.

"In some respects, health care services appear to be the same in the HMO as in other health care organizations—the same basic health professionals and ancillary personnel are present in an institutional setting similar to the acute hospital, nurses provide similar services and fulfill the needs of patients, and physicians' roles remain conceptually unchanged except for payment patterns. In contrast, the HMO provides an opportunity for nurses to broaden the traditional definition of nursing. That is, by creating a potential setting for more fulfilling work, the HMO presents a context for the unrestricted utilization of nurses' diverse skills" (Smith 1980, p. 54). An important question is whether managed care organizations enable nurses to meet their needs for autonomy, self-actualization, and esteem. In the studies reported by Smith (1980, 1981), HMOs appeared to be positively fulfilling their potential for meeting both the personal goals of nurses and the goals of the organization.

Illustrations

The position of the nurse working in a managed care organization is unique, even though the same functions and role are performed in other settings. This uniqueness results from the linked financing and delivery structure of the managed care organization, which increases the nurse's authority when interacting with other professionals and with the patient. Although persuasion and motivation are still important features of interactions within a managed care organization, the nurse enters the interaction process from a position of strong authority. As a result, the nurse can have greater influence on the performance and outcomes of the system.

As this section of the book has indicated, nurses perform many functions and fulfill many roles in managed care organizations. Perhaps one of the most widely identified roles is that of the primary care provider. Many managed care organizations, especially staff and group model HMOs, employ nurse practitioners to work independently in terms of their practice sites, with physicians providing backup coverage. These nurse practitioners provide well-baby care, well-woman care, and treat minor acute care illnesses such as sore throats and earaches. In many instances, members are encouraged to make appointments with the nurse practitioner as their primary care provider. Nurse practitioners are supported by the managed care organizations, and the quality of care provided is stressed to prevent them from being viewed as simply a lower-cost alternative.

Managed care organizations with Medicare risk contracts also use nurse practitioners extensively to serve that population. For example, when a new Medicare member enrolls in the plan, the nurse practitioner begins to develop a data base by initiating a visit with the member to do an initial history and physical exam. During this health assessment, the nurse practitioner can determine if the member is fairly healthy and does not need to see a physician immediately, or if the member has multiple health problems requiring immediate physician intervention.

If the member does not need immediate attention, the nurse practitioner may review the history and physical exam findings with the physician for corroboration of findings or identification of areas missed and to schedule a follow-up visit if needed. If the member has medical problems that need immediate attention, an appointment is made and the physician assesses the patient and initiates treatment. The nurse practitioner usually continues to monitor the patient for compliance with the prescribed regimen and to evaluate the effectiveness of the treatment. In addition, the nurse practitioner provides patient education in terms of dietary requirements, exercise program, necessity of adequate rest and sleep, and the other aspects that are critical in maintaining a certain level of health.

In other situations, the nurse practitioner, because of advanced training, actually runs the urgent care clinics during the day, treating those patients presenting with problems within his or her expertise and facilitating immediate access to physicians for problems outside that expertise. If the managed care plan is located in a state that licenses nurse practitioners as independent providers with prescribing powers, then the nurse practitioner can prescribe antibiotics for such conditions as ear infections, laryngitis, or vaginal infections. In terms of the urgent care setting, face-to-face access to a provider versus telephone consultations may substantially enhance the patient's satisfaction with the system.

Nurses in managed care organizations are also significantly involved in case management. For example, many newly diagnosed cancer patients are assigned a case manager to work with their primary care physician. The case manager begins working with the patient and the physician at the time of the initial diagnosis.

If the initial diagnosis is made during a hospitalization, then the nurse case manager would be responsible for working with the discharge planning components, coordinating necessary referrals to oncologists, radiation oncologists, and others and coordinating necessary home health services. The nurse case manager would also provide education for the patient and family in terms of what to expect.

When the patient is discharged from the hospital, the case manager will continue to stay in touch with the patient and family. This monitoring may initially consist of nothing more than a phone call during the first week after discharge to ask: "How are things going? Did your home health nurse show up? Have you gotten the equipment you need? Did you get your appointments with oncology? Radiation? Have you been seen?" Based on how quickly the disease progresses, the case manager may only stay in touch with that patient once a month.

If the patient begins to deteriorate, the case manager's role becomes more involved. He or she ensures that any equipment needed in the home is obtained, that needed increases in home health and homemaker services are provided, and, if necessary, exceptions to plan benefits are procured if it can be documented that these services will prevent more expensive institutionalization or utilization of resources.

By visiting the patient in the home, the nurse case manager is in a position to say to the physician, "This patient is getting dehydrated, we need to start some IVs," or "The pain is not really being kept under control, we need to look at stronger pain medication or at more invasive methods of controlling pain" (for example, going from oral pain medications to subcutaneous medications, epidurals, or IV pain medications). Although much of the case manager's contact with the patient may be by telephone, personal contact is maintained to ensure that appropriate access to other services is obtained and that benefit exceptions are extended if necessary. Because of extensive involvement with the patient and family, the case manager is in a position to help them when hospice care is needed.

The case manager is also usually involved in helping the patient and family decide whether the patient should stay at home to die or become institionalized, and then making those wishes happen. Often this is a benefit exception issue because, under these conditions, plans often do not cover institutionalization. However, the case manager is in a position to know if the family is going to be able to handle death in the home and, if not, to minimize the expenses associated with placing the patient in an institution when death approaches. For such interactions to occur, however, the managed care organization and the case manager cannot keep members at arm's length. The nurse must be involved as both a coordinator of care and a resource allocator. Obviously, the nurse functions as a patient advocate throughout this process.

Increasingly in managed care organizations, nurses are filling the role of patient educator. For example, when the managed care organization has a diabetic nurse educator, then all diabetic patients are referred to him or her. The diabetic nurse educator does all the initial teaching relative to their disease and what it means; how to care for themselves and the use of insulin or oral medications. Whereas most new diabetics in managed care organizations are scheduled to see a dietician, the nurse educator is in a position to continue to reinforce the teaching over time, especially since most managed care organizations do not cover more than two or three visits to a dietician for the newly diagnosed patient.

In addition, nurses in managed care organizations often provide wellness education; smoking cessation education; education on healthy lifestyles—role of diet and exercise; and prenatal care and everything relative to maternity, childbirth, and new infants. Traditionally, most prenatal education has occurred in hospitals, but the managed care organization assumes more responsibility and provides a nurse educator so that members receive all the desired information relative to childbirth education. The managed care organization provides more control over the entire process, and nurses play a vital role in ensuring quality and managing resources within this system.

Case Studies

The following case studies reinforce the concepts presented in the book and illustrate many of the functions and activities nurses perform in managed care settings. Although individual case studies may emphasize a specific function or activity, additional functions and activities are integrated in the problem-solving approach.

The first five case studies follow a common format consisting of six major components: 1) problem statement; 2) background; 3) role of the nurse; 4) problem-solving approach; 5) outcome; and 6) implications. The last two case studies follow a different format, but include the concepts in the major components of the first five case studies. These seven case studies are not meant to represent comprehensive documentation of the particular problem addressed; rather, they are intended to identify a problem and then illustrate how nurses, in collaboration with others, have approached the problem and the results of their interventions.

#1: Infant Patient

Problem Statement: An infant girl has multiple medical problems and the plan must determine whom to involve in managing the care of the infant; what types of services and setting are most appropriate for the infant; and when benefit exceptions should be pursued. Incorporating the preferences of the family increases the complexity of the decision-making process.

Background: An infant girl with multiple congenital abnormalities has been in an acute care hospital for $3^1/2$ months during this last readmission. Her medical problems include the following:

- profound mental retardation
- spina bifida
- respiratory problems requiring tracheostomy
- tube feedings.

The infant is subject to frequent periods of apnea and requires constant total care. She is the couple's only child. The father is totally deaf and cannot hear the apnea monitor alarm. The HMO's benefit plan only covers intermittent nursing care services, not constant care. To complicate matters, the state, which frequently pays for private-duty nursing at home for such infants, has no funds to cover new cases this fiscal year. The only pediatric skilled nursing facility in the state currently has a two-year waiting period for admission, and the mother will not even consider applying for a position on the waiting list. The mother repeatedly demands that the child be brought home. In addition, the state does not cover services provided in another state.

In deriving a satisfactory solution to this complex situation, the following parties were involved: the plan's pediatric continuing care RN (CCRN), a plan social worker (who is a pediatric specialist); the infant's pediatrician; the primary family practice physician; a home medical equipment supplier; a hospital social worker; members of a home health team; an agency development center; the pediatric nursing staff of therapists; the resident physician; a state department of health care manager; and the child's parents. The plan's utilization review manager and the continuing care supervisor were also involved because of benefit policy/coverage issues. Decisions to make benefit exceptions were approved by the chief and deputy medical directors.

Role of the Nurse: It is the policy of the plan that its neonatal CCRN review and follow all problem newborns. This child had been placed in the plan's selective case management program at birth by the CCRN. The neonatal CCRN reviewed the admission and identified the level of care required during the neonatal admission. At that time, the CCRN developed the first discharge plan, ordered special home-care medical equipment, and arranged for parental instruction in caring for the infant at home. A plan social worker conducted home visits and followed the patient's family until the first readmission to the hospital. The child's condition continued to deteriorate at home, and after repeated admissions for pneumonia secondary to aspiration, a tracheostomy was performed and feeding tubes were inserted. The child's mother was still determined to care for the child at home.

During the last hospitalization, the pediatric CCRN reviewed the admission and hospital stay and was in constant communication with the child's pediatrician and primary care physician. She monitored the child's condition and communicated with the child's mother several times a week at the hospital. When the child's condition began to stabilize, the CCRN organized a discharge team and prepared an initial care plan for taking the infant home again. With the help of the plan social worker, who had been involved with the family since the infant's birth, a number of care options were evaluated and several cost analyses performed. The CCRN negotiated with vendors for equipment and services, preventing delays and barriers to fulfilling the discharge plan. Immediately after the discharge, the CCRN visited the mother and infant in the home. When the child was readmitted briefly, the CCRN again managed the care.

Problem-Solving Approach: This case was reviewed regularly at the continuing care/social service weekly meeting during which all problem inpatients are discussed. The chief and deputy medical directors were aware of the options being considered and approved pursuit of an intensive home-care program. The CCRN reported that the parents were adamant about caring for the child at home. The CCRN felt this child was very fragile, but since the mother would not consider the pediatric skilled nursing facility, the only other option available was continued hospitalization. During the extended re-admission, the mother lived at the Ronald McDonald House and family life was nonexistent. The mother participated in the child's care, but refused to take the child home without a guarantee that a minimum of eight hours per day of private-duty nursing would be covered and paid for by the plan as long as the child was at home.

The plan CCRN and social worker, with the approval of the plan pediatrician who directed the child's care during the hospital admission, organized a discharge planning meeting at the hospital. Before the meeting, the chief medical director and deputy medical director responsible for utilization management had tentatively approved payment for private-duty pediatric nurse coverage as part of the home-care plan. The state department of health nurse care manager was invited because the state was expected to pay for services when funding again became available.

A needs assessment and discharge plan were developed by the plan CCRN and social worker, and were signed by the child's pediatrician for submission to management. At the same time, a cost analysis was prepared by the CCRN, social worker, and utilization review manager, who compared the cost of home care to the cost of maintaining the child in the hospital. These documents were presented to the chief medical director by the deputy medical director and the care plan was approved. The plan's policies require such assessment and cost analysis before any extraordinary case management plan can be approved.

Before the child was discharged from the hospital, the mother spent a weekend at the hospital caring for her using the medical equipment provided by the durable medical equipment supplier chosen by the plan. The CCRN made arrangements for some of the medical equipment and electrical rewiring of the house to be donated or paid for by Medicaid, since the plan does not cover such benefits. A special visual device to allow the deaf father to see rather than hear the alarms on the apnea monitor was also installed by the plan.

Outcome: The child is still at home, but the plan has had to increase the nursing time to twelve hours a day. The child has only been in the hospital for four days since discharge under this plan. The mother is still anxious to keep the child at home. The plan now provides periodic respite care at a pediatric skilled nursing facility, and is attempting to get the parents to agree to place the child on the waiting list at the skilled nursing facility in the event that the family can no longer care for the baby at home. Considering placement of the child in a facility is a very sensitive issue for the parents, but the strain of keeping the child at home is apparent: In just two months, the parents are now physically and emotionally stressed.

Implications: During the management of caring for this patient, the plan discovered several important aspects of its coverage and structure:

1. The plan learned that contract vendors must clearly understand that orders for equipment changes must come only from the plan. In this case, for example, when the severely hearing-impaired father complained that the vibrations from the compressor interfered with his sleep, the vendor installed an expensive outside unit that doubled the cost of oxygen without notifying the plan. The plan then had to negotiate with the family and vendor to use the new equipment only at night in order to reduce the costs of this option. Also, Medicaid was required to pay for the new equipment since the plan's durable medical equipment benefit limit had already been exceeded.

2. The plan learned that regular home visits by the primary care physician, the CCRN, and the social worker were essential to the success of the care plan. The CCRN visited several times during the first week at home.

3. The parents refused counseling after the child was born. The plan social worker, who was part of the discharge planning team, has an MSW and is certified to provide counseling. In cases such as this one, assessment of family members by a competent mental health professional is essential. Although counseling cannot be mandated, the family should be strongly encouraged to accept counseling to help them manage the severe stresses this situation places on them individually and on their marriage.

4. It is essential that an alternative plan be developed in case the home plan does not work. The mother has visited the pediatric skilled nursing facility, which has a two-year waiting period for residence. This skilled nursing facility does accept children for respite care and has been known to accelerate the waiting period for humanitarian reasons. The plan CCRN arranged for and accompanied the mother on this visit.

5. Time limits for benefit exceptions must be built into the plan. The initial eight hours of RN time were promised for as long as the child was at home and in need of services. The additional four hours were provided on a month-to-month basis. When state funds become available, the state is expected to pay for the four-hour differential.

6. The case should be reviewed frequently, and written status reports should be required. The plan CCRN must continue as case manager, not the agency nurse.

7. The plan should make the patient's parents part of the care process from the beginning and insist that they participate in the care at the hospital. In any home care plan, the parents are

the primary caregivers, not the plan or the contract nurses. The parents must understand this and accept the responsibility or the care plan will not work.

8. Long-term plans should be made. It should not be assumed that a child or adult is being sent home to improve or die after a short interval.

9. The plan must know the cost of the proposed care plan before promising anything to the family. The cost analysis should be in writing and plan management should understand the financial obligations before the CCRN promises the family anything.

10. A periodic review of actual costs should be conducted to determine if the vendors are billing and being paid correctly.

11. The plan should consider a written "contract" with the family for home services. In this case, the contract has never been signed because of the uncertainty about the benefit of such a contract to the plan. The plan has given the family a written care plan detailing the equipment, services, and payment source.

12. If a support group is available, the parents, especially the mother, can often benefit from association with people in similar circumstances who have suffered the same feelings of guilt, isolation, fatigue, and desperation.

13. Families such as this—with a child who is so seriously impaired that she will require total care with frequent admissions to hospitals for all of her predictably short life—must be given the opportunity and the information necessary to make choices about the means used to continue that life. This is an area in which the CCRN is uniquely placed to assess the family's evolving attitudes, beliefs, hopes, and expectations about the child. In the plan's experience, the CCRN can help the family make their concerns known to the physicians.

#2: The Return of Tuberculosis

Problem Statement: From 1953 through 1984, the number of reported cases of tuberculosis declined about 5 percent annually. Then, a slow increase started in the number of reported cases so that by 1988 there were more than 22,000 cases and 1,600 related deaths reported annually.

In 1987, the federal government established the Advisory Committee for Elimination of TB (ACET), and charged it with devising a strategy for eradication of the disease by the year 2010. About 25 percent of those exposed to TB actually become infected; of these, 10 percent develop clinically active tuberculosis at some point in their lives. The TB skin test should be used to screen all individuals exposed, especially those at greatest risk: young, old, and those with weakened immune systems from malnutrition, alcohol and drug abuse, chronic illness, and HIV infection. Reactions between 5 and 15 millimeters in duration generally represent function/exposure. Izoniazid (INH) therapy decreases the risk of active disease by 60 to 80 percent. Of importance in the plan's patient population is the increase in the proportion of cases in the nonwhites (in 1953, nonwhites accounted for 24 percent of the TB population; in 1988, this population accounted for 65 percent). Foreign-born individuals account for 20 percent of the case rate. Minority groups account for more than 80 percent of childhood cases of active disease. However, for all groups, the highest disease rate is in the elderly. (See Dowling 1991 and Dowdle 1989.)

Background: The patient is a nineteen-year-old black male college student, a basketball player, a nonsmoker, and was healthy until November 1990, when he presented with lower respiratory tract infection symptoms (fevers to 102 degrees, chills, sweats, nonproductive cough, malaise, anorexia, and a ten-pound weight loss). His chest x-ray (CXR) noted a left lower lobe infiltrate. He improved somewhat on Erythromycin, but continued to experience exercise intolerance. A purifed protein derivative (PPD) and candida implanted were positive. Eventually, he was started on INH, Rifampin, and Pyridoxine. He developed Rifampin sensitivity and was switched to Ethambutol. He is currently on pyrazinamide (PZA) and INH. This patient lives with both parents and one sister who had received INH prophylaxis from 1986 to 1987.

Role of the Nurse: There are numerous roles for the nurse in the management of this case, as there are many more aspects than the individual patient. To begin, a plan nurse is the first contact the patient usually has via the triage system. The nurse makes the decision regarding appropriate appointments for the patient. For this patient, it is the nurse who also interacts with the system and the patient to ensure that diagnostic screening is completed (lab work, x-rays, PPD, mumps/candida antigen placement) and that compliance with medical regimen occurs.

The family also required TB screening and the father subsequently was started on INH prophylaxis. The basketball team and coach required screening, and were informed and referred, as needed, to the local department of health.

Throughout the course of this patient's adjustment to his medication, he required close follow-up. As previously mentioned, his medication must be taken for an extended period of time, and success rates with compliance are tied to the direct, continuous interaction with the nurse.

Problem-Solving Approach: The problem-solving approach for this case is multilevel. In sequence, the patient, his family, and his team required care. Close collaboration between doctors and nursing staff were required. This individual case, however, points to the larger issue of screening and preventive therapy. Because of the location of the plan's centers and the multi-ethnic/racial population, all staff should be aware and screen appropriately. Once the decision is made to treat (if active) or prophylax, dose follow-up is mandatory.

Outcome: Enforced adherence to protocol is essential, as is aggressive screening and follow-up. The seed beds of tuberculosis are really those who are infected, particularly those in whom the bacillus multiply. PPD skin test reactions focus attention and efforts where the benefit-risk ratio is greatest. In many large metropolitan areas, the seed beds of TB are the foreign-born, the elderly, certain impoverished minority populations, the homeless, and those with HIV infection.

Implications: Quality care and service provision requires teamwork. For preventive and screening processes to achieve successful results, intensive follow-up is required over an extended period of time. The plan must commit sufficient resources, especially nurses' time, to foster successful compliance.

#3: Chemical Dependency

Problem Statement: The following medical management problem involves multiple decisions by several of the affected parties, including:

- benefit coverage and determination of eligibility for a treatment not covered in the HMO's benefit plan purchased by the patient's employer
- comparison of treatment capabilities between contracting and noncontracting facilities
- investigation of allegations of poorly qualified staff employed at a plan-contracting facility (the allegations have been made public)
- Assessment of appropriate level of care (inpatient versus outpatient)
- ethical issues of recommending treatment within the network (cognizant of the quality of care allegations) when the patient has refused to consider switching physicians (to contracting providers); and recommending chemical dependency (CD) treatment given previous history of treatment outcomes and poor prognosis

- assessment of the importance of continuity of present provider/ patient relationships given that previous care was received at the nonparticipating facility.

Background: A fifty-four-year-old male is three months post inpatient treatment for chemical dependency (he has a thirty-year history of alcohol abuse with multiple inpatient stays in the last fifteen years). In the past three months, he has continued with outpatient treatment and has been fairly successful with abstinence. He also has poorly controlled diabetes, mild hypertension, and has recently been diagnosed with cirrhosis. He lives alone in the inner city with no telephone.

Today, he presented to his attending physician with lethargy and admitted to having had "a couple of drinks" in the past few days. His blood sugar was 641 (recently ranging from 389 to 676). His liver function was found to be severely compromised.

The attending physician was concerned with the status of the diabetes, as well as the potential indication of a liver transplant for the patient. The physician is requesting admission to the noncontracted chemical dependency facility for inpatient treatment, as well as diabetes management, since previous treatment had occurred at that facility (after much patient reluctance, but ultimately good relationships were established), and the facility is capable of treating all diagnoses.

The patient became eligible for health plan benefits in the last thirty days; however, the mental health benefit rider was not purchased by the patient's employer. The patient had a difficult time admitting his chemical dependency to others during his last hospitalization; he claims he was not aware that his health benefit did not include coverage for mental health/chemical dependency treatment.

According to plan policies, the health plan medical director analyzes all issues relative to any case. Previously, the medical director has tended to make prudent, appropriate decisions.

The patient's physician is a general practitioner who is extremely concerned with the patient's diabetes and cirrhosis status. This physician has a very busy office practice; therefore, he delegates authorization of hospitalizations to the receiving hospital. Consequently, limited information is available to the health plan for authorization of services in this scenario. The general practitioner, however, feels that disruption of the current relationship between patient and treating psychiatrist would not be harmful.

The treating psychiatrist is not on staff at the contracted facility. He contacted the health plan medical director in an effort to persuade him to authorize treatment at the noncontracted facility. The psychiatrist questioned the plan's goals in managing care, making the accusation that the plan permits technicalities to dominate its review decisions, not concern for the patient's health and welfare. He challenged the plan's selection of a contracted facility, reminding the medical director that the contracted facility has had negative publicity regarding its employment of poorly qualified staff.

The nonparticipating hospital admissions representative contacted the health plan and requested authorization for the admission via the attending physician's direction. This representative threatened to go to the media if the admission was not approved at the nonparticipating facility as there is widespread awareness of the staff qualification issues at the health plan's contracted facility. The admissions representative was very persistent in obtaining the authorization for treatment.

Role of the Nurse: The nurse interacts with all necessary parties to access complete case information in a timely fashion. In this case, additional medical information was needed from the attending physician's office due to the limited information available from the hospital requesting authorization. An assessment was made by the nurse case manager as to the medical appropriateness of the proposed treatment plan.

Before approval of the proposed plan could be given, a determination of the patient's coverage status had to be made—the benefits interpreted. To avoid setting precedents for the plan, legal resources had to be consulted regarding the plan's policy related to providing benefits outside of the benefit contract.

In terms of quality assurance and risk management, previous public allegations of the employment of unqualified staff at the contracted facility necessitated an investigation of the facts and outcome of those allegations. A legal opinion also had to be obtained regarding continued use of this facility, especially for this patient, given the aggression of the admissions representative of the nonparticipating hospital.

The nurse performed the role of provider liaison in conjunction with and/or secondary to the medical director. All medical information, benefit determination, and quality assurance findings are routinely presented to the medical director to ensure that appropriate decisions can be made.

The nurse also functions as a patient advocate and a health educator. At the appropriate time—when the patient was medically stable—the nurse contacted the patient to inform him about the coverage provided in his benefit contract, including the fact that not all services are automatically purchased through an employer-sponsored benefit contract.

Problem-Solving Approach: In terms of benefit interpretation and coverage issues, the following activities were undertaken:

1. verification of the patient's health plan membership
2. review and certification of coverage for requested services
3. consultation with legal resources regarding the plan's liability for providing medically necessary, uncovered benefits (in excess of the contract)
4. discussion with the employer about the potential ramifications of providing a benefit in excess of the current contract (while maintaining patient confidentiality) relative to the employee's claim that he was not informed that the mental health benefit was not available
5. review of findings with the medical director.

In terms of possible utilization of out-of-network services for this patient, the following steps were performed:

1. contacted the attending physician and the nonparticipating psychiatrist to discuss issues related to the previous quality allegations made against the contracted facility
2. determined the level of services required by the patient
3. ascertained whether the participating facility could provide the necessary treatment at acceptable standards of care
4. researched the option of obtaining the contracted rate at the nonparticipating facility.

To meet the needs of the patient appropriately, effectively, and efficiently, alternative treatment plans were developed and analyzed. The plan identified and assessed alternative options to inpatient treatment, reviewed the proposed treatment plan against the plan's established criteria for care, and presented the case findings and treatment options to the medical director for peer review. The plan also assisted the patient in exploring resources available for funding the services.

The plan also explored the options available for non-covered services and identified community resources available to the patient after discharge from the hospital.

The plan also encouraged the patient to utilize community resources such as Alcoholics Anonymous and explored the availability of employer-sponsored support services through the employee assistance program.

Outcome: In the management of this patient's care, an extra-contractual decision was made to provide the benefit in the contracted facility (the patient agreed since he was not financially responsible). An investigation of the allegations regarding employment of poorly qualified staff at the contracted facility found the information to be outdated. The employees involved in the allegation were no longer employed.

The health plan's medical director did not succumb to peer pressure regarding the quality allegations made against the contracted facility; and denied the admission to the non-participating facility.

The patient was treated for all of the diagnosed conditions simultaneously during inpatient treatment. A new psychiatrist with admitting privileges at the contracted facility was assigned the case; and disruption of the original relationship between the nonparticipating psychiatrist and the patient was not harmful.

In addition, the patient was reeducated regarding his benefit plan contract. The employer agreed to extracontractual payment for this particular stay at the health plan's contracted rate due to the fact that the employee was uninformed about his health insurance policy and chemical dependency stay costs per day were less than acute medical costs per day. The employer agreed to reevaluate his position on exclusion of all mental health benefits for employees. Legal implications and negative public relations were avoided since a treatment option was approved that did not compromise the patient's medical status.

Implications: Several policies and protocols of the plan were reinforced, but the need for others and for flexibility in designing appropriate care plans were identified. The following issues were especially relevant in this case:

- The importance of coordinating all activities with the medical director and his or her involvement at each step in the process were reinforced.
- The need for reevaluation by the health plan of the provider credentialing process was identified. It is essential that the process accommodate the collection and receipt of quality-of-care information in a more timely fashion.
- The ability to negotiate an agreement with the employer was exercised to explore the options available to make more expansive benefits available to the employee while controlling costs.

#4: Ventilator Patient

Problem Statement: The management of this patient was complicated by conditions at home and benefit limitations of the plan. A number of policies and issues were presented during the provision of care to this patient.

Background: A non-Medicare-age HMO patient remained in the plan-owned hospital for eight months with end-stage chronic obstructive pulmonary disease (COPD). She was ventilator-dependent at night and had suffered several bouts of respiratory infections. There were no nursing homes close to her home to meet her care needs. Although she had end-stage COPD, her prognosis was unclear. Being ventilator-dependent, she could live for a year or for several years. If she stayed in the hospital, the costs would continue to climb.

Upon entering the case, the hospital liaison nurse discovered that the patient wanted to go home. In addition, the nurse found that the HMO wanted the patient to go home, if possible. At the start, the liaison nurse found a series of obstacles delaying the discharge of the patient. A major obstacle was the fact that the patient lived in an older house that would have to be rewired to handle the ventilator and supporting medical equipment.

Although the patient's son also lived in the home, he was only willing to help out a few hours a day with her care. Complications also set in because the plan's durable medical equipment benefit did not cover the type of respiratory equipment needed by the patient. In addition, the patient had not applied for any state assistance (Medicaid) in the past.

Role of the Nurse: The hospital liaison nurse coordinated the patient's discharge. The nurse facilitated the development of an alternative care plan, obtained additional benefits and resources, and was an advocate for the patient.

Problem-Solving Approach: There was a series of meetings with the hospital nursing staff and a discharge planner. A social worker also became involved in the process. The social worker and the hospital liaison nurse started a Medicaid application for state assistance and a Social Security Disability application that could lead to Medicare funding for this patient. The discharge planner helped mobilize the hospital personnel that would be required to implement the proposed care plan. These critical personnel included the hospital's plan physicians, staff nurses, respiratory therapists, and hospital administration. The hospital liaison nurse's job was to alert and help orient the home health staff to the possibility of managing a ventilator-dependent patient at home.

Inpatient respiratory therapists held a series of training sessions for the patient, her family, and home health staff. Volunteers were recruited and the house was rewired. The state agreed to pay for some attendant care under a special program called COPES. Hospital administration agreed to make exceptions and pay for additional equipment and additional private help.

As the date for discharge approached, the coordination of activities was under the control of the hospital liaison nurse. A ventilator had to be obtained for home use and intensive training had to be set up for all those involved in her care. The initial schedule to cover her twenty-four-hour nursing care needs was developed and different funding sources were identified. The entire discharge planning process took about six weeks.

Outcome: The patient remained at home for two years. The liaison nurse continuously remained in contact with the patient during this time. Attendant requirements changed and schedules had to be adjusted. There was a hearing before an administrative law judge regarding the state's obligations in this case.

During these two years, the patient's son was in a serious car accident, which drastically changed the provision of services to meet the care needs of the patient. The patient had two short hospitalizations for respiratory infections during these two years.

Even with these obstacles, most participants were pleased with the arrangements. The HMO realized significant cost savings, the patient frequently expressed pleasure at being able to stay at home, and it helped give the HMO new direction in its home health services program.

Implications: As a result of this case, there were major changes made to the HMO's medical care policies. Standing contracts were arranged with private agencies to provide for attendant and respite care in selected cases. Protocols were developed for home ventilator care and new pilot programs were started to try to manage different types of cases at home with a combination of home health and attendant care. It seems apparent that the liaison nurse will continue to have a vital role in the expanding role of home health care in the future.

#5: AIDS Patient

Problem Statement: The medical management of an AIDS patient presented plan management with a number of significant care, cost, and ethical issues. Among these were the following:

- reevaluation of the plan's benefit coverage for treatments considered experimental or investigational
- reassessment of the scope of the treatment capabilities within the plan network to determine the appropriateness of out-of-plan network referral
- reevaluation of mechanisms for determining appropriate level of care (inpatient versus outpatient or home health services)
- consideration of the ethical issue of treatment resources being allocated to a terminally ill patient.

Background: A 29-year-old male presents to the emergency room with nausea and vomiting for six days, and blurred vision in his left eye and loss of vision in his right eye for the past ten days. There is copious drainage from both eyes. The patient had been diagnosed as HIV-positive eight days before his emergency room admittance. At time of admission, the patient was diagnosed as having AIDS-related cytomegalovirus (CMV) retinitis.

The patient's primary care physician has referred the patient to a participating infectious diseases specialist for assessment. The specialist recommends referral to a nonparticipating infectious diseases specialist with subspecialty expertise in treatment of AIDS-related CMV retinitis. The nonparticipating specialist indicates that immediate hospitalization is necessary at the nonparticipating university hospital in order to initiate treatment with a trial drug. The patient needs a one- to two-week inpatient stay for dosage regulation and thereafter will require four days of outpatient IV therapy per week for life. It is believed that without treatment the patient will incur permanent blindness within four to ten days. The long-term prognosis for the patient is very poor.

The patient's objective is to maintain his eyesight at any cost. The patient is irrational and emotionally overwhelmed following his recent AIDS diagnosis.

The plan medical director tends to be ineffective in fulfilling the medical director's role of benefits interpreter, provider liaison, and physician consultant in cases like this. The medical director's previous reluctance to make decisions in this type of case appear to be associated with lack of experience and expertise in the role of medical director and in this specific type of case. The primary care physician, a family practitioner, was a cooperative participating provider whose priority was to support any treatment protocol that might benefit his patient. The primary care physician expressed concern regarding his lack of experience and qualifications, as well as time constraints, in his ability to manage this case effectively.

The first referral physician, a participating infectious diseases specialist, was a cooperative physician who, after diagnosing the patient with CMV retinitis, is very concerned that aggressive, available treatment be rendered immediately. The second referral physician, a nonparticipating infectious diseases specialist, was not on staff at any of the plan hospital facilities. This physician indicated that the patient was an appropriate candidate for the drug trial, but also displayed substantial hostility in regard to treatment coverage issues and plan staff involvement in the case management process.

A contracted plan home health agency was interested in assessing the opportunities for alternative care in the treatment plan. However, the home health agency has indicated that it currently does not have experienced staff who could manage the drug therapy or CMV retinitis.

Role of the Nurse: In the role of case manager, the nurse was an information-gatherer and researcher. The nurse gathered pertinent case information from each of the parties involved in order to assess the appropriateness of the recommended treatment and to judge whether or not more cost-effective care alternatives were feasible. In this case, research needed to be done to determine possible in-network care alternatives, optional treatment plans, and the coverage status of requested treatment.

In the role of benefits interpreter, the nurse needed to determine the plan coverage status of the trial drug treatment. A recommendation needed to be made as to the necessity of utilizing nonparticipating providers or offering an in-network alternative. In addition, the nurse consulted with legal resources on coverage policy issues and obtained expert opinions from resources that supported the plan's coverage decision.

The nurse performed the provider liaison role secondary to or in the absence of the medical director. The nurse discussed plan findings and possible coverage alternatives with involved providers in order to obtain "buy-in" to the treatment plan of choice.

As an educator and patient advocate, the nurse contacted the patient to discuss the proposed case management and to provide information on additional community resources available for financial and emotional support. The nurse reeducated the patient on the coverage options provided in his plan contract.

Problem-Solving Approach: In terms of benefit interpretation and coverage issues, the plan reviewed the member's certificate of coverage and obtained drug status information from the Food and Drug Administration (FDA)—the drug is not FDA approved. The plan obtained local expert professional opinion on the proposed treatment plan, contacted a national resource expert to discuss the treatment plan and alternatives, and obtained the coverage position of local and national competitors.

In addition, the plan consulted with legal resources on the above findings and reviewed the findings with the medical director.

With respect to out-of-network referral, the nurse did the following in collaboration with other members of the patient's care team:

- researched in-plan network options in terms of physicians
- researched in-plan facility options and determined the level of service requirements for providing the treatment option by

obtaining temporary physician privileges for a nonparticipating physician
- explored financial arrangements with the nonparticipating physician and hospital.

In developing alternative treatment plans, the plan assessed acuity and skilled care needs of the patient's care; consulted with the expert physician on the possible treatment combination options—inpatient, outpatient, and home care; proposed the preferred level of treatment alternatives to the medical director; and obtained "buy-in" on the proposed alternative treatment plan from the patient's primary care physician, the referral physicians, and the patient.

In managing the allocation of resources, the nurse: identified alternative sources of funding, educated the member of available community resources for support and care, encouraged the member and his support system to explore the hospice concept in the management of the terminal condition, and determined the most cost-effective means of providing the necessary care.

Outcomes: In developing a care plan for the patient, coverage for experimental treatment was specifically excluded in the plan contract. The plan agreed, however, to cover the physician and hospital services associated with the experimental treatment. The drug costs for the trial drug were covered with outside research funds. Legal experts supported the coverage of such care because the economic implications of setting a coverage precedent in this rare case did not outweigh the political and liability risks associated with a denial of coverage.

Approval from the plan CEO for the proposed treatment was obtained in the absence of the medical director's decision to cover treatment costs other than drug costs. Also, the plan approved referral for nonparticipating physician services because the necessary subspecialty physician expertise was not available in the network. The nonparticipating physicians were reimbursed at the reasonable and customary rate in the community. The plan also obtained temporary physician privileges at the participating hospital facility for the nonparticipating infectious diseases specialist.

In providing the treatment, a five-day inpatient stay for dosage regulation at the participating hospital facility was approved. During the patient's five-day stay, the staff from the home health agency obtained trial drug therapy training and also managed the necessary home IV therapy for ten days after hospital discharge. Subsequently, the patient received ongoing IV therapy on an outpatient basis.

The patient joined an AIDS support group and also requested from the plan information on hospice program coverage. By modifying the benefit coverage for this patient, the plan avoided possible negative public reactions that could have been incurred if treatment had not been covered and a threatened media blitz regarding poor quality care had occurred.

Implications: This case illustrated the following to the plan:

- the importance of having an effective coordinator research and conduct follow-up reviews concerning final determinations and case outcomes
- the need to weigh various factors in the decision making process, for example, medical appropriateness, legal liability, public relations, and economics
- a need for improved training and education of the medical director as a decision maker and provider liaison in a managed care role
- the importance of having a supportive primary care physician maintaining control of patient management rather than deferring it to a consulting physician
- the need to have effective member benefit education at the time of enrollment and on an ongoing basis
- the importance of managing care to achieve appropriate lower-cost treatment alternatives
- the need for the development of a medical director training program
- a need to evaluate the primary care physician's incentives with respect to the ongoing management of a patient's care following referral to a specialist.

#6: Newborn Patient

Documentation: Sarah was born on August 8, 1989, after a normal pregnancy and swift delivery. Life has been a struggle ever since. She arrived with Walker-Warburg syndrome, cataracts, brain malfunction, muscular dystrophy, a urinary tract infection, pneumonia, and soon needed a gastrostomy tube and a shunt. Sarah was the only child of parents whose careers required them to work out of the home.

On the first day following Sarah's birth, the continuing care RN introduced herself to the family and began working with Sarah and her parents. By September 7, the CCRN had arranged for the baby to be discharged to the family at home; this, despite the perinatologist's skepticism that neither the parents nor the infant could cope. Armed with a kangaroo pump, a sleep apnea monitor, two well-trained parents, and the confidence of the CCRN, young Sarah went home.

The family wasn't abandoned, however. Nurses from the continuing care program visited twice a day every day for months, and an LPN stayed for twelve hours during the night-time hours. Care has gradually tapered off in the past two years. It has been nearly a year since Sarah's last hospitalization and she is stable. The continuing care nurses arranged for the family to apply for Medicaid and a private foundation to pick up coverage as plan benefits for some services expired. All durable medical equipment has been left with the family.

Now, the CCRN checks with the family on a monthly basis to be sure the situation is still stable. Sarah's parents have been delighted with the CCRN, the pediatrician, and the health plan. They love having their baby home and have achieved a certain sense of normalcy in their lives.

Questions:
1. What circumstances combined to make this a success story?
2. What roles have the nurses played?
3. What skills did the continuing care nurse need to pull this off?
4. Was the pediatrician a factor in the success of this case?

#7: Leukemia Patient

Documentation: Betty Lou was a member of Phoenix Health, a non-profit HMO. She had been covered by the plan for eight years through her husband's job at city hall, but had seldom needed to call on her coverage even with three young children. In fact, up until two years ago she would have described herself as boringly healthy.

Things changed quickly. Betty Lou's mild asthma became markedly more acute and she sought treatment for a duodenal ulcer, all within about a six-month period in 1989. These were manageable conditions from which she rebounded. Even her occasional cocaine abuse wasn't causing her any apparent problems. Then, in August 1990, came the real blow: She was diagnosed with lymphocytic leukemia (Burkette's type).

Betty Lou's physicians started her on a course of Vincristine Cytosine and Leucovorin. Predictably, on September 12, she was evaluated as a candidate for a bone marrow transplant, and two brothers were found to qualify as potential donors. However, two weeks later it was discovered that Betty Lou's husband was HIV-positive as a result of an IV drug habit. Her initial HIV screen (Eliza test) in early October was positive. No consultants could answer the $64 question: Had the leukemia altered the blood tests to result in a false positive?

At the end of October, Betty Lou was accepted for the transplant program, but her Western Bloch test also came back positive for HIV. The ethical, legal, and medical questioning and evaluations began, and the discussions were often heated. The medical staff was divided and the board was not clear about which way to turn. Finally, the medical director ruled in early November that Betty Lou's transplant should proceed and she was admitted to the hospital. The plan's case management department was then notified and a nurse was assigned to work with Betty Lou.

Events moved rapidly. On November 4, Betty Lou became disenchanted with the entire process and discharged herself from the hospital against medical advice. She refused all home health care and soon developed shingles and pleural effusion. On December 1, she developed pneumocystis pneumonia and was placed on AZT and Pentamidine, as was her husband. On December 10, she entered the hospital for the bone marrow transplant, but she left the institution against medical advice once again. She returned on December 26 and the transplant was performed. Betty Lou never left the hospital and died on April 3, 1991.

Questions:

1. What roles might nurses have played to improve the situation?
2. What about timing? Were nurse case managers involved at the right time?
3. Was the case well-handled and was the transplant appropriate?
4. The children still belong to the HMO's plan. Is there a nursing role here?

Future Directions

The nursing profession is changing rapidly in response to turbulent societal and health services environments. The need for change is expected to intensify as environmental forces continue to change.

One factor significantly affecting nursing is the changing age composition of the population. An increasing proportion of the population today is age sixty-five or older; by 2050, it is projected that approximately one-third of the population will be sixty-five or older (Kutzka 1985). Many of these individuals will suffer chronic medical problems requiring long-term assistance. "Such factors as a highly mobile population, decreased family sizes, and multiple family members in the work place, may diminish the ability of family members to provide primary support services" (Waite 1989, p. 17). In addition, as family members live to the age of eighty-five and beyond, the "younger" family members are in their sixties and seventies and developing medical problems of their own. All of this increases the need for medical and social support assistance.

Closely related to the changing age structure of the population is the changing pattern of diseases. At the turn of the century, the three leading causes of death in the United States were: 1) pneumonia and influenza; 2) tuberculosis; and 3) diarrhea, enteritis, and ulceration of intestines. By the 1990s, the three leading causes of death were: 1) diseases of heart; 2) malignant neoplasms; and 3) cerebrovascular accidents (National Center for Health Statistics, 1990). As the disease patterns of the population shift from acute illnesses to chronic illnesses, the focus of the medical field must shift from cure to maintenance. The need to understand the complexities of the physical, psychological, and social requirements of the patients' illnesses exceeds the need to understand the biological origins of the disease. Increasingly, the focus of the health care system will be on managing and stabilizing illness rather than curing disease.

As the health care industry accounts for an ever-increasing proportion of the gross national product of this country, efforts will increase to limit the amount of resources going to that sector. The increased emphasis on cost control will stimulate creativity in alternatives for delivering quality care. Increasingly, emphasis will be placed on managing the resources utilized by the industry and attention will focus on providing cost-efficient and cost-effective health care services. Increasingly, the industry and, therefore, health professionals will be held accountable for the benefits of their services relative to the costs. Technology adoption will increasingly be examined in terms of need, costs, and outcomes.

In response to these pressures, the health care industry will increasingly look to various strategies for managing resources and utilization of services. As efforts are made to control costs, strategies must also be adopted to ensure that quality of care is not adversely affected and that access to care is not unduly restricted. All of these efforts are directed at changing the culture of the organization and of the health care delivery system. "Included in these cultural changes are the mandating of outpatient surgery for many operations, same-day admission surgery, hospices, formularies, nonduplication of services, generic prescription drugs, home health care, step-down units, nursing homes as alternatives to long-term hospitalization, and copayments and deductibles. . . . Each of these methods seek to change the behavior of the provider and/ or the patient" (Wenzel 1991, p. 372).

A factor limiting nursing's ability to respond fully to these pressures and demands from the health care system is the persistent shortage of nurses. Strategies to alter the manner in which care is delivered are increasingly affected by the difficulties encountered in recruiting and retaining nurses. "When one of the most critical resources of any industry is in short supply, the implications are felt throughout the organizations within that industry. ... As direct and indirect purchasers of nursing services, managed care entities must become increasingly involved in how institutional providers deal with this shortage" (Johnson 1991, p. 43). As managed care organizations struggle to contain costs, this shortage of nurses increases the cost of this resource, potentially altering the way nurses will be utilized in the future delivery of health care services.

According to St. Amand (1988), the following events can be expected in the future:

- utilization review of all ambulatory care
- outpatient certification
- utilization review in home health
- profiles of physician office practices
- expected outcomes and time lines on care
- more capitated pricing or per diems for care given
- increased networking and linkages with systems
- nonexclusive agreements
- more contracted care
- more predetermined pricing by volume
- increased independent medical case reviews (medical audits)
- increased centralized care management (p 17).

These events are all directed at managing care in one way or another. The role of nursing in accomplishing these activities will be enhanced, especially if the shortage of nurses can be overcome. Controlling the intensity and the frequency of the utilization of health care services in the delivery of quality care will be the focus of the health care system in the foreseeable future.

References

Albrecht, K. 1979. *Stress and the manager.* Englewood Cliffs, NJ: Prentice-Hall, Inc.

American Nurses Association. 1980. *Nursing: A social policy statement.* Kansas City, MO: Author.

American Nurses Association. 1988. *Nursing case management.* Kansas City, MO: Author.

Araujo, M.D., and J.T. Jurkovic. 1984. "The role of nursing in quality assurance." In J. Pena, A. Haffner, B. Rosen and D. Light. *Hospital quality assurance: risk management and program evaluation.* Rockville, MD: Aspen Systems, pp. 219–236.

Arnold, T.H. 1981. Quality assurance issues in health education: Maximizing patient satisfaction. *GHAA Proceedings* 31: 206–212.

Bailey, A., K. Hallam, Karyn, and K. Hurst. 1987. Triage on trial. *Nursing Times* 83(44): 65–66.

Ball, M.J., J.V. Douglas, R.I. O'Desky, and J.W. Albright. 1991. *Healthcare information management systems: A practical guide.* New York: Springer-Verlag.

Benson, D.S. and P.G. Townes. 1990. *Excellence in ambulatory care.* San Francisco: Jossey-Bass Publishers.

Boland, P. 1991. *Making managed healthcare work: A practical guide to strategies and solutions.* New York: McGraw-Hill, Inc.

Boyd, Steven, et al. 1991. Professional nursing roles: The reintegration of patient teaching. *Journal of Nursing Staff Development* 7(2): 88–90.

Brill, E.L., and D.F. Kilts. 1986. *Foundations for nursing* (2nd ed.). Norwalk, CT: Appleton-Century-Crofts.

Bunsey, S., M. DeFazio, L.L. Pierce, and S. Jones. 1991. Nurse managers: Role expectations and job satisfaction. *Applied Nursing Research* 4(1): 7–13.

Carmel, S., I. Yakubovich, L. Zwanger, and T. Zalteman. 1988. Nurses' autonomy and job satisfaction. *Social Sciences and Medicine* 26: 1103–1107.

Cline, B. 1990. Case management, organizational models and administrative methods. *Caring* 9(3): 14–18.

Coleman, J.R. and E. Hagan. Collaborative practice: Case managers and home care agency nurses. *The Case Manager* 2(4): 64–72.

Coleman, J.R. 1990. HMOs and individual case management. *The Case Manager* 1(3): 55–61.

Council of Primary Health Care Nurse Practitioners. 1985. *The scope of practice of the primary health care nurse practitioner.* Kansas City, MO: American Nurses Association.

Cowan, D.H. 1984. *Preferred provider organizations: Planning, structure, and operation.* Rockville, MD: Aspen Systems.

Crosby, P.B. 1980. *Quality is free: The art of making quality certain.* New York: New American Library.

Culp, B., N.D. Goemaere, and M.E. Miller. 1985. Risk management: An integral part of quality assurance. In C.G. Meisenheimer, *Quality assurance: A complete guide to effective programs.* Rockville, MD: Aspen Systems, pp. 169–192.

Daniels, K. 1988. Will nurses control care at home? *Home Healthcare Nurse* 6(2): 18–23.

Davis, B.V. 1989. How do you incorporate patient education into everyday practice? *HMO Practice* 4(2): 54–56.

Davis, C.K. 1990. Financing of health care and its impact on nursing. In J.C. McCloskey and H.K. Grace. *Current issues in nursing.* St. Louis, MO: The C.V. Mosby Company, pp. 352–356.

del Togno-Armanasco, V., G.S. Olivas and S. Harter. 1989. Developing an integrated nursing case management model. *Nursing Management* 20(10): 26–29.

Derdiarian, A.K. 1991. Effects of using a nursing model-based assessment instrument on quality of nursing care. *Nursing Administration Quarterly* 15(3): 1–16.

Dowdle, W.R. 1989. A strategic plan for the elimination of TB in the USA. *MMWR* 38(Supplement 3): 1–25.

Dowling, P. 1991. Return of TB: Screening and preventive therapy. *American Family Physician* 43(2): 457–466.

Duran, G.S. 1980. On the scene, risk management. *Nursing Administration Quarterly* 5(1): 19–36.

Ebers, D.L., and L. Smith. 1989. A vision for the future: Quality principles for health maintenance organizations. *GHAA Proceedings* 39: 75–113.

Eck, S.A., and N.H. Ryan. 1990. The era of counterbalancing technology in pediatric nursing. In J.C. McCloskey and H.K. Grace, *Current issues in nursing.* (3rd ed.). St. Louis, MO: The C.V. Mosby Company.

Ersoz, C.J., and N. Forney. 1991. St. Clair Hospital: The quality enhancement process. In P. Boland, *Making managed healthcare work.* Gaithersburg, MD: Aspen Systems, pp. 417–420.

Fagin, C.M. (1982). Nursing as an alternative to high-cost care. *American Journal of Nursing* 56–60.

Faherty, B. 1990. Case management, the latest buzzword: What it is and what it isn't. *Caring* 9(7): 20–22.

Findlay, S. October 30, 1989. Looking over the doctor's shoulder. *U.S. News and World Report* 110(44).

Fondiller, S.H. 1991. How case management is changing the picture. *American Journal of Nursing* 91(1): 64–80.

Friel, M., and C.B. Tehan. 1982. Counteracting burn-out for the hospice caregiver. In E.A. McConnell. *Burnout in the nursing profession: Coping strategies, causes, and costs.* St. Louis, MO: The C.V. Mosby Company, pp. 150–159.

Geiger, J., and J.S. Davit. 1988. Self-image and job satisfaction in varied settings. *Nursing Management* 19(12): 50–58.

Germain, C.B. 1984. *Social work practice in health care: An ecological perspective.* New York: The Free Press.

Gillies, D.A., M. Franklin, and D.A. Child. 1990. Relationship between organizational climate and job satisfaction of nursing personnel. *Nursing Administration Quarterly* 14(4): 15–22.

Gluck, J. 1980. Primary care: The extension of primary nursing. In K. Zander, *Primary nursing: Development and management.* Rockville, MD: Aspen Systems, pp. 281–293.

Group Health Cooperative of Puget Sound. 1984. *Nurses' guide to telephone triage and health care.* Pacific Palisades, CA: Nurseco Inc.

Hackman, J.R., and J.L. Suttle. 1977. *Improving life at work.* Santa Monica, CA: Goodyear Publishing Co.

Harper, L. 1976. Developing and evaluating a patient education program. In *Patient Education.* New York: National League for Nursing.

Hartman, M. 1976. An historical perspective on quality assurance. In *Pathways to Quality Care.* New York: National League for Nursing, pp. 1–5.

Health Insurance Association of America. 1990. *Source book of health insurance data.* Washington, DC: Author.

Henderson, V. 1966. *The nature of nursing.* New York: MacMillan.

Holt, F.M. 1990. Managed care and the clinical nurse specialist. *Clinical Nurse Specialist* 4(1): 27–29.

Johnson, C. 1991. Supply and demand in the labor market for registered nurses: The implications for managed care organizations.'' In *GHAA Annual Meeting Proceedings.* New York: Group Health Association of America: 41–58.

Keane, C.B. 1986. *Essentials of medical-surgical nursing* (2nd ed.). Philadelphia: W.B. Saunders Company.

Knollmeuller, R.N. 1989. Case management: What's in a name? *Nursing Management* 20(10): 38–42.

Kohnke, M.F. 1980. The nurse as advocate. *American Journal of Nursing* 80(11): 2039–2040.

Kohnke, M.F. 1982. *Advocacy: Risk and reality.* St. Louis, MO: The C.V. Mosby Company.

Kongstvedt, P. 1989. *The managed health care handbook.* Rockville, MD: Aspen Systems.

Kralovec, O.J.; C.A. Huttner, and M.D. Dixon. 1991. The application of total quality management concepts in a service-line cardiovascular program. *Nursing Administration Quarterly* 15(2): 1–8.

Kutzka, E. 1985. *Social and health policies on aging.* Racine, WI: Johnson Foundation.

LaBar, C. and R.C. McKibbin. 1986. *New organizational models and financial arrangements for nursing services.* Kansas City, MO: American Nurses Association.

Langenfield, M. 1988. Role expectations of nursing managers. *Nursing Management* 19(6): 78–79.

Like, R.C. 1988. Primary care case management: A family physician's perspective. *Quarterly Review Bulletin* 14(6): 175–178.

McCloskey, J.C., and H.K. Grace. 1990. *Current issues in nursing.* St. Louis, MO: The C.V. Mosby Company.

McConnell, E.A. 1982. *Burnout in the nursing profession: Coping strategies, causes, and costs.* St. Louis, MO: The C.V. Mosby Company.

McKenzie, C.B., N.G. Torkelson, and M.A. Holt. 1989. Care and cost: Nursing case management improves both. *Nursing Management* 20(10): 30–34.

Meisenheimer, C.G. 1985. *Quality assurance: A complete guide to effective programs.* Rockville, MD: Aspen Publications.

Mills, M.E. and O'Keefe, S. 1991. Computerization: A challenge to nursing administration. In M.J. Ball et al. *Healthcare information management systems: A practical guide.* New York: Springer-Verlag, pp. 103–113.

Mowry, M.M., and R.A. Korpman. 1989. *Managing health care costs, quality and technology: Product line strategies for nursing.* Rockville, MD: Aspen Systems.

National Center for Health Statistics. 1990. *Vital statistics of the United States.* Washington, DC: U.S. Government Printing Office.

O'Connor, C.T. 1990. Patient education with a purpose. *Journal of Nursing Staff Development* 6(3): 145–147.

O'Hare, P.A., and M.A. Terry. 1988. *Discharge planning: Strategies for assuring continuity of care.* Rockville, MD: Aspen Systems.

Porter, L.W. et al. 1974. Organizational commitment, job satisfaction and turnover among psychiatric technicians. *Journal of Applied Psychology* 59: 603–609.

Radecki, S.E., R.E. Neville, and R.A. Girard. 1989. Telephone patient management by primary care physicians. *Medical Care* 27(8): 817–822.

Record, J. et al. 1981. *Primary care staffing in 1990.* New York: Springer.

Redman, B.K. 1980. *The process of patient teaching in nursing* (4th ed.). St. Louis, MO: The C.V. Mosby Company.

Rowland, H.S., and B.L. Rowland. 1985. *Nursing administration handbook.* (2nd ed.). Rockville, MD: Aspen Systems.

Sabins, J.E., L. Forrow, and N. Daniels. 1991. Clarifying the concept of medical necessity. In *GHAA Annual Meeting Proceedings*. New York: Group Health Association of America. pp. 693–708.

Salmon, M.E. and P. Vanderbush. 1990. Leadership and change in public and community health nursing today: The essential intervention. In J.C. McCloskey and H.K. Grace. *Current issues in nursing*. (3rd ed.). St. Louis, MO: C.V. Mosby Company, pp. 187–193.

Scherer, J.C. 1986. *Introductory medical-surgical nursing* (4th ed.). Philadelphia: J.B. Lippincott Company.

Schlesinger, E.G. 1985. *Health care social work practice: Concepts and strategies*. St. Louis, MO: Time Mirror/Mosby College Publishing.

Schuler, H.J. 1991. The strategic management of quality. *Nursing Administration Quarterly* 15(2): 53–58.

Scott, M.P., and K.P. Packard. 1990. *Telephone assessment with protocols for nursing practice*. Philadelphia: W.B. Saunders Company.

Scully, G.L., and A.O. Nichols. 1990. Case management: Compilation of definitions. *The Case Manager* 45: 42–43.

Shipske, G. 1982. An overview of case management supervision. *Caring*: 5–10.

Sliefert, M.K. 1990. Quality control: Professional or institutional responsibility? In J.C. McCloskey and H.K. Grace. *Current Issues in Nursing* (3rd ed.). St. Louis, MO: The C.V. Mosby Company.

Smith, H.L. 1980. Quality of working life in a health maintenance organization: Comparison of medical and ancillary personnel. *Journal of Ambulatory Care Management* 3(4): 37–47.

Smith, H.L. 1981. Nurses' quality of working life in an HMO. *Nursing Research* 30(1): 54–58.

Sox, H.C. 1979. Quality of patient care by nurse practitioners and physician's assistants: A ten-year perspective. *Annals of Internal Medicine* 91: 459–468.

St. Amand, L.V. 1988. Managed care: Fitting pieces into the puzzle. *Home Healthcare Nursing* 6(2): 14–17.

Stewart, M.L. 1988. Nurse-midwifery service as a cost-containment measure in a managed health-care plan. *Medical Interface* 2(11): 8–10.

Stillwaggon, C.A. 1989. The impact of nurse managed care on the cost of nurse practice and nurse satisfaction. *Journal of Nursing Administration* 19(11): 21–27.

Stone, C.L., and K. Krebs. 1990. The use of utilization review nurses to decrease reimbursement denials. *Home Healthcare Nurse* 8(3): 13–17.

Tischler, G.L. 1990. Utilization management and the quality of care. *Hospital and Community Psychiatry* 41(10): 1099–1102.

Tranbarger, R.E. 1991. Nurses and computers: At the point of care. In M. Ball et al. *Healthcare information management systems: A practical guide*. New York: Springer-Verlag.

Van Kempen, S. 1979. The nurse as client advocate. In Clark and Shea. *Management in nursing—A vital link in the health care system*. New York: McGraw-Hill Book Co.

Waite, R.M. 1985. The driving forces for change. In McCarthy. *Nursing's vital signs: Shaping the profession for the 1990s*. Battle Creek, MI: W.K. Kellogg Foundation.

Walker, M., and D.L. Wong. 1991. A battle plan for patients in pain. *American Journal of Nursing* 91(6): 32–36.

Weil, M., and J.M. Karls. 1985. Historical origins and recent developments. in M. Weil et al. (Eds). *Case management in human service practice.* San Francisco: Jossey-Bass.

Weiner, J.P., D.M. Steinwachs, and J.W. Williamson. 1986. Nurse practitioners and physician assistant practices in three HMOs: Implications for future U.S. health manpower needs. *American Journal of Public Health* 76(5): 507–511.

Wenzel, F.J. 1991. Managed care. In A. Ross, S. Williams, and E. Schafer. *Ambulatory care management* (2nd ed.). Albany, NY: Delmar Publishers, Inc., pp. 370–382.

Winder, P.G. 1990. Successful triage in ambulatory care. *American Journal of Nursing* 90(3): 28F–28G.

Wiseman, S.J. 1990. Patient advocacy: The essence of perioperative nursing in ambulatory surgery. *Association of Operating Room Nurses Journal* 51(3): 754–762.

Yura, H. 1973. *The nursing process* (2nd ed.). New York: Appleton-Century-Crofts.

Zander, K. 1990. Case management: A golden opportunity for whom? In J.C. McCloskey and H.K. Grace. *Current issues in nursing.* (3rd ed.). St. Louis, MO: The C.V. Mosby Company.

Acknowledgment

The following individuals contributed materials utilized in the development of the case studies discussed on pp. 86–87.

JoAnn Appleyard, RN
   RUSH-ANCHOR Organization for Health Maintenance
John Coleman, Ph.D.
   Quality Managed Care, Inc.
Muriel H. Constantine, RN
   Rhode Island Group Health Association
Paul Ehrlich, RN
   Group Health Cooperative of Puget Sound
Mary Enger, RN
   United HealthCare Corporation
Carolee Fauth-Brooks, RN
   CHP
Elizabeth Gandara, RN
   Kaiser-Permanente Center for Health Research
Janet E. Gyselinck, RN
   Care Choices
Marcia K. Hock, RN
   Harvard Community Health Plan
Linda W. Johnson, RN
   QualChoice
Pattie Carroll Kearns, RN, MA
   HealthShield
LeAnn Lee, RN
   United HealthCare Corporation
Elizabeth L. Scheer, RN, MN
   Ochsner Health Plan
Janet Stallmeyer, RN, MSN
   Care Management, Inc.
Patricia White, RN
   Michael Reese Health Plan Inc.

SECTION THREE

THE FUTURE OF
MANAGED CARE AND NURSING

Managed care organizations and nursing are at important junctures in their histories. The challenges facing the managed care industry and nursing are similar, and nursing should take advantage of this convergence to further the provision of compassionate, caring, cost-effective health care services. Clearly, nurses are in an excellent position to take advantage of the changes occurring in the health care system. The education and professional philosophy of nursing makes this profession especially qualified to make the changes needed to move managed care organizations from a paradigm of medicine to a paradigm of health.

As internal and external pressures intensify the necessity for change in the health care system, the futures of managed care and nursing will increasingly be interlocked. As managed care organizations struggle to provide quality services under greater resource constraints, tremendous opportunities will be created for nurses, as employees and as private contractors. To capitalize on these opportunities, nurses must expand and enhance their intrapreneurial and entrepreneurial knowledge and skills. Nurses must increasingly be willing to take business risks as they provide cost-effective, quality health care management for their patients.

The continued demand for cost-effective health care solutions rather than medical solutions will push more buyers (governments, employers, individuals) into managed care arrangements (Brisk 1986). With this increased demand for managed care solutions, a growth in current managed care options can be expected, along with the introduction of more innovative programs into the market. This shifting paradigm will place increasing challenges on nursing to provide the necessary inputs and on the profession to adapt to these pressures or be replaced by other professionals who can and will change to meet the new pressures. For nurses, the increasing shift to managed health care creates tremendous opportunities to acquire new roles, gain more practice autonomy, become economically independent, and increase their intrapreneurial and entrepreneurial skills. Today's nurses have more opportunity than ever to capitalize on the turmoil and chaos surrounding the current health care system (Sweeney and Witt 1990).

Trends Increasing Opportunities

According to Maraldo (1991), the growing trend in managed care will provide increasing opportunities for nurses to gain prominence in health care delivery and to be the mainstream providers of care. Three trends are especially working in nursing's favor and will create tremendous opportunities for nurses to use their cost-saving, quality-care-providing capacity.

First, in the shift from a predominantly inpatient, hospital-oriented system to a community-based ambulatory system of managed care, nursing is the profession of practitioners best suited to manage a patient's care. Across delivery settings—as patient advocate, patient educator, and practitioner in caring for the chronically ill—nursing will emerge as the mainstream provider of coordinated care in the 1990s. In essence, nurses will be the new gatekeepers of the health care system. While this is already happening in managed care organizations, corporations and insurers have recently begun employing nurses to determine how resources should be optimally allocated to serve the patient best. These entities are increasingly using nurses to answer the questions: Is the treatment plan appropriate? Is it effective? Is the setting appropriate? Is there adequate follow-up? These types of questions are at the foundation of the role of the nurse in utilization review and case management in managed care (Maraldo 1991).

Second, purchasers of health care are increasingly turning their attention to value received from services purchased and used, not just price. As purchasers become more prudent buyers of health care services, they will be looking for additional valuable alternatives to the traditional service delivery systems. In the new value-conscious health care climate, nurses will have the opportunity to compete directly with other care providers to offer the best package of health care services at the best price. Nurses and nurse-run provider organizations will develop independent preferred provider arrangements; however, they will also be the predominant means for contracting health services among HMOs, PPOs, insurance carriers, and self-insured employers and their covered populations (Maraldo 1991). To be successful, nurses and nursing organizations are going to have to be able to demonstrate that the value of the services they provide is greater relative to price than services from other providers.

Third, as the health care system moves toward some form of national guaranteed, basic access system (even if coverage remains fragmented), increasing restrictions and regulations will be put in place to limit and control access to specific points of health care services; to coordinate care among a number of points of service; and to manage the use, cost, and quality of care at all these points. With managed care as a centerpiece of these controls, the nursing profession can play a greater role as mainstream providers of care (Maraldo 1991). As government payment increases, the need to control costs will also increase. This trend is closely related to the trends associated with seeking maximum value for resources used and the prudent buyer concept of payers.

These three trends will create more opportunities for nurses as employees of managed care organizations, as well as more opportunities for nurses to form group practices and private individual practices to provide services independently. As Drucker (1985) pointed out, a change in industry structure offers exceptional opportunities for innovation and entrepreneurial pursuits; and, the current structure of the health care industry is certainly changing rapidly.

Intrapreneurial Nursing Opportunities

Concept of Intrapreneurship

The term "intrapreneur" was coined by Gifford Pinchot to describe entrepreneurial individuals inside an organization. According to Pinchot (1985), an intrapreneur is "any of the 'dreamers who do.' Those who take hands-on responsibility for creating innovation of any kind within an organization. The intrapreneur may be the creator or inventor but is always the dreamer who figures out how to turn an idea into a profitable reality" (p. ix). These individuals are the agents and catalysts of change. An intrapreneur possesses intense desires to make things work better and has the necessary ability and willingness to take risks within the organization to convert these ideas into profitable (financial and quality, value-added) realities. In the health care industry, profitable is not just viewed as an improved financial condition, but any improvement (quality, structure, productivity) in the health care delivery system. "Intrapreneurs are self-determined goal setters who often take the initiative to do things no one asked them to do" (Pinchot 1985, p. 49). As individuals very familiar with how activities in an organization are performed, they are in an excellent position to identify changes that will improve the performance of these activities. Nurses, therefore, are in positions to function extremely well as intrapreneurs.

Intrapreneuring Nursing Opportunities

Because of their number and direct contact with the health care consumer, nurses are key participants in meeting the challenges of the emerging health care system. To maximize the contributions of nursing in this new environment, health care organizations must encourage nurses to exercise their creative potential. "The nurse intrapreneur is one who creates innovation within the health care organization through the introduction of a new product, a new service, or simply a new way of doing something" (Manion 1990, p. 2). To survive and prosper in the future, health care organizations are going to need to encourage, support, and reward innovation among their employees.

Major societal changes are having significant impacts on the organization and operation of the health care delivery system. These changes are presenting numerous opportunities for nurses to expand their roles within these organizations and to make major contributions to the field. Manion (1990) identified eight major societal trends affecting the health care industry:

- shift from industrial society to an information society
- shift in technology from high-tech to high-touch
- shift from short-term to long-term
- shift from centralization to decentralization
- shift from institutions to self-help
- shift from a representative to a participative democracy
- shift from hierarchies to networks
- shift from either/or choices to multiple options.

These trends are having substantial effects on the health care industry. As the industry struggles to adapt to these changes, nurses are in an excellent position to influence the responses to them and to increase their innovative and creative roles in the industry. Nurses employed in health care organizations are in a key position to influence those organizations positively.

The health care industry has experienced a tremendous explosion in technology and knowledge in recent times. This rapid growth has led to a corresponding need for individuals to be able to process and communicate enormous amounts of information in reaching clinical and practice decisions. "The nurse is at the hub of virtually every health care organization, and by virtue of a strong generalist educational preparation, is a key information worker. Instead of defining the nursing role by sorting through and focusing on the tasks the nurse does, a focus on the critical role the nurse plays in gathering, processing, and acting on information will be the basis of future opportunities" (Manion 1990, p. 140).

To maximize the opportunities for nursing in this information-driven environment, nurses must become assertive in converting ideas and concepts into action. As a central component in the provision of health services, nurses assemble and process tremendous amounts of information (clinical, process, practice, and structure) and therefore have enormous opportunities to be creative and innovative in the organization.

Because of the structure and incentives inherent in managed care organizations, the ability to process and communicate information is especially critical. As managed care organizations attempt to control access to various points of service, nurses' knowledge about the implications of those controls will be crucial. Because of nursing's role throughout the organization, nurses are increasingly functioning as the gatekeepers to the system. Nursing therefore has the opportunity to be creative and innovative in collecting, processing, and communicating information to help managed care organizations make appropriate, cost-effective access decisions.

The current restrictive-resource environment is forcing organizations to modify their attitudes and actions surrounding their human resources. Under the historical unlimited resources mentality, health care organizations tended to view their employees as interchangeable, replaceable inputs. Turnover among employees was not viewed as detrimental to the organization since a new supply was readily available and the organization did not expect its employees to do more than perform designated tasks. Now, organizations are looking for long-term commitment from their staff and are encouraging them to become innovators within the system. For the organization to survive and prosper, internal improvements in the way tasks are performed and services provided are essential (Manion 1990). Employees are excellent sources of ideas for improving the operations of the organization because of their detailed, intimate knowledge of the functions of the organization.

Nurses are in an excellent position to provide leadership in these areas and to identify new and better ways of providing services to the clients. As managed care organizations are increasingly forced to compete for limited resources, nurses can offer better, cost-effective ways of meeting the needs of the clients.

As organizations increasingly recognize the value of nurses in the decision-making process, changes are being made in the way nurses and nursing activities are structured. "The degree of control a nurse feels over practice issues, scheduling, and work place management has been recognized as a key issue in nurse retention" (Manion 1990, p. 143). To take advantage of the opportunities to participate in management decisions, nurses have to be willing to change and to consider critically new ideas and approaches to problem solving. To maximize the opportunities available, nurses need to learn new skills in business and market analysis. Even if the nurse has no intention of leaving the organization and establishing a private practice, an understanding of business and economics is important in meeting the challenges of the new environment (Batra 1991). If nursing is unwilling or unable to change and adapt to the new marketplace pressures, then nurses will be replaced with professionals who can and will adapt.

For nurses to perform optimally within the organization, they must be given (or take) sufficient freedom to function as intrapreneurs. The organization must be willing to recognize the value of the services provided by nursing and to encourage and reward nurses for making changes that improve the cost-effective delivery of quality health care services.

In developing intrapreneurial models within the organizations, certain common elements appear to be critical. "The elements that appear essential to the success of such models are autonomy in nursing practice, decentralized responsibility for decision making, and compensation practices consistent with a professional approach to delivering nursing services" (York and Fecteau 1987, p. 166). In the current turbulent environment, nursing must seize the opportunities to increase its independence, practice control, and decision-making powers within the organizations.

Individual Advantages

Nurses can seize innovative, creative opportunities in the marketplace without leaving an organization and establishing their own independent practice. Individual initiative can also be used to create innovations within an organization. Manion (1990) identified six intrapreneurial advantages for the individual who remains with an organization. First, remaining with an organization means that the organization shares the risks surrounding the new idea or product and, usually, can afford to invest more resources in the development and marketing of the innovation. Second, the organization provides access to its numerous contacts in marketing the new product or service. Third, "as an employee within the organization, the nurse intrapreneur has access to a vast network of people who can be trusted to answer questions, offer assistance, and help make the innovation successful" (p. 3). Fourth, many organizations offer internal educational opportunities as well as support for external professional development; in addition, the intrapreneurial process can lead to professional growth as new and different skills are developed. Fifth, professional satisfaction is increased as the nurse intrapreneur affects the system and thereby the welfare of a large number of people. Sixth, involvement in a large organization provides opportunities for feedback, recognition, and rewards: "The *esprit de corps* which results from successful innovation within an organization is very energizing, generating a strong, positive, and enabling atmosphere within the work place'' (p. 5). Nurse intrapreneurs can use these advantages to enhance their professional growth and the role of nursing in the health care delivery system.

Institutional Advantages

Intrapreneurship also offers numerous advantages to the organization. To survive in the current turbulent environment, organizations must be innovative and creative. An excellent source of innovation and creativity comes from the talents and expertise of the employees working within the organization. To tap those talents, ''an environment must be created where ideas are sought from all levels of the organization, and where those employees with good ideas are rewarded'' (Manion 1990, p. 5). The organization, and the individual, can benefit financially and qualitatively from the innovations of intrapreneurs. These innovations can also provide the organization with a competitive edge in the market place. The professional and personal satisfaction intrapreneurs experience enables the organization to attract and retain them, and they, in turn, tend to be more productive (Manion 1990).

An organization where there is a cooperation among workers, loyalty and commitment to the best interests of the organization, and excellent employee relations is one that promotes team spirit. The presence of team spirit differentiates intrapreneurs from entrepreneurs. Nurses have valued teamwork through the decades. Nurses are now demanding more decision making power within the health care team so the resources are available for them to provide patient care. Hospitals that are responsive and that provide essentials (such as support for innovation and change, fair compensation practices, and autonomy over practice) have greater likelihood of gaining a higher perceived degree of supportiveness among the people employed within the organization (Boyar and Martinson 1990, p. 30).

The supportive environment of the organization can lead to the development of new products and services by the intrapreneurs, which can generate revenue for the organization. Intrapreneurs' creativity can also result in new ideas for solving problems and improving the efficiency with which resources are used in providing services. This increase in productivity is also financially beneficial to the organization.

Necessary Skills

Although nurses involved in intrapreneurial practices are all different, they tend to exhibit a fairly consistent set of characteristics and traits. The degree to which each of these characteristics is necessary depends to a large extent on the climate of the organization: The more supportive the organization, the lower the requirement for the nurse to possess and utilize these basic skills and characteristics. Manion (1990) has identified certain personal, leadership, and business skills as necessary for success as an intrapreneur.

Personal. "Personal skills directly related to a nurse intrapreneur's success include, but are not limited to, assertiveness, negotiation, risk taking, and time management" (Manion 1990, p. 34). To be successful, the nurse intrapreneur must know when to be personally and professionally assertive. It is not sufficient for the nurse to be assertive in clinical and practice situations; he or she must also be assertive in dealing with organizational problems or situations. Because of the professional role nurses perform throughout the organization, these individuals are in an excellent position to identify where and why problems occur and to offer creative, innovative solutions—if they can convey their impressions and ideas in an assertive way without becoming aggressive.

To be influential within an organization, an individual must become involved in activities such as task forces and committees where problems and strategies are discussed and decisions are made. Although involvement in these activities detract, at least temporarily, from direct patient care, the solutions proposed and implemented may have a substantial impact on overall service delivery, affecting many more clients than a single nurse could affect simply by providing direct patient care. "The very act of assertion presupposes that the individual believes in himself/herself and embodies self-confidence and a high level of self-esteem, has the ability to identify the basic human rights involved in the situation, and has confidence in these rights and will act on them" (Manion 1990, p. 36). Again, the basic education and philosophy of nursing instills and reinforces these beliefs in basic human rights.

In order for people to convince others that what they have to contribute to the situation or to the organization is valuable, they must hold themselves in high esteem. The nurse must be convinced that his or her actions and opinions make a difference and can influence decisions and solve problems. "Organizational norms are strong influences on self-esteem. Throughout our lives, we are judged in large part by how we measure up to unwritten 'rules' of behavior—some of which are constructive, while others are destructive'' (Manion 1990, p. 37). Unless these organizational norms support the power of the individual in solving problems and affecting decisions, they can quickly undermine the intrapreneurial efforts of nurses, creating dissatisfaction and draining the creative efforts of the staff. "Nurses have a unique contribution to make to health care organizations, and must speak up and take an active role in guiding the changes that are coming in the future. If the nurse believes in his/her value to the organization and understands his/her own special qualities, this will increase confidence in making intrapreneurial contributions. The nurse must value his/her nursing practice and unique professional contributions, or the self-esteem needed for intrapreneurship may not be present" (Manion 1990, p. 38). The education and philosophy of nursing gives nurses many special qualities, abilities, and skills to make major contributions to the restructuring of the health care delivery system. To be effective, however, nurses must be assertive in convincing others of the value of their contributions.

To be successful as an intrapreneur requires the nurse to be a skillful negotiator. "Negotiation occurs when people exchange ideas with the intention of changing relationships, or when people confer for agreement. If there is a need to be met, there is a potential negotiating situation" (Manion 1990, p. 39). To foster cooperation among coworkers and gain administrative support in the organization, negotiations must be approached from a win-win position. Antagonistic approaches to negotiation must be avoided and the problem must be approached and solved in a positive direction for all parties involved. Innovations in an organization are quickly stifled if participants are concerned about "getting even" for previous actions or winning at any price. To be successful, the nurse intrapreneur must have the support of others in the organization.

Being a nurse intrapreneur involves risk—by definition, intrapreneurs effect change and change always has an element of uncertainty and risk. The key to taking risks is to minimize the uncontrollable features of that uncertainty (Drucker 1985). There is risk in proposing new ideas, products, or services because being new implies that the outcome cannot be known with certainty. However, the potential losses associated with the unknown can be minimized by carefully identifying possible results and their implications. Risk can never by entirely eliminated, but being willing to take a calculated, moderate chance is the only way to grow professionally.

In balancing his or her personal and professional life, the nurse intrapreneur must manage time successfully. Time management requires the skills of planning, setting priorities, being personally organized, and overcoming the tendency to procrastinate (Manion

1990). Planning involves establishing objectives and developing strategies for achieving those objectives. In outlining the steps to be taken in reaching the objective, the importance of each task needs to be determined so that critical activities can be undertaken first. To ensure that the important tasks are accomplished, a systematic, organized approach to estimating the time required for each task and possible barriers to completion must be prepared. Any project has certain unpleasant or boring aspects; however, the completion of these tasks are critical to achieving an objective, so they must be dealt with and not postponed until they threaten the success of the entire project (Manion 1990). The successful nurse intrapreneur develops the personal skills of assertion, negotiation, risk taking, and time management.

Leadership.   Whenever the innovations of a nurse intrapreneur require the efforts of other people, leadership skills are important. "Key leadership skills include communicating a vision, gathering input from others, facilitating a group process, leading a meeting, coaching coworkers, motivating others, delegating tasks or responsibilities, and coordinating the efforts of others (Manion 1990, p. 34). Although the nurse intrapreneur may initially visualize the innovation to be completed, most new products or services require the efforts of others. The nurse intrapreneur must be able to motivate others to be involved in the development of the innovation and able to delegate tasks and responsibilities to others in order to accomplish the necessary activities. The nurse intrapreneur must also be skilled in facilitating group effort. To be successful, the nurse intrapreneur must be able to lead others, not just manage their work (Manion 1990).

Business.   Once an idea for a new product or service has been conceptualized, the next step is to plan how it can be implemented. In order to convince others in the organization of the value of the idea, the nurse intrapreneur must be able to describe the product or service and explain the reasons why it is needed. To be administratively accept-able, the service or product should benefit the organization. The determination of these benefits often requires an analysis of the existing market for substitute or competitive products along with an explanation of the resources required to develop and produce it. The identification and presentation of a comprehensive list of potential requirement (personnel, equipment, supplies, support, etc.) is critical in convincing others of the merit of the idea. "All goals, objectives, and tasks of the proposal culminate in a financial plan. The entire plan now must be translated into dollars and cents" (Manion 1990, p. 109). It may not be necessary for the nurse intrapreneur to possess the skills to perform each of these business planning activities, but it is important that he or she recognizes the importance of performance. In many organizations, the necessary expertise can be obtained from others (an advantage of remaining with an organization instead of establishing an independent practice). However, the expertise to complete the tasks may not be necessary, although the nurse must understand enough about the process to communicate effectively with the experts in other areas.

"Writing a winning business plan takes effort. It also requires creativity, ambition, and commitment. The planning, data analysis, and writing that are required offer significant challenges for the nurse intrapreneur. Today's cost-conscious health care field requires that nurses sharpen their skills in these areas" (Manion 1990, p. 116).

In order for nursing to take full advantage of the many opportunities created by the changes in the health care industry, nurses must have the skills to provide innovative solutions to problems. Although opportunities to expand the role of nursing are extensive, these same opportunities can become threats if nurses do not possess the necessary skills and motivation to capitalize on them. As precarious as the future of many health care organizations is, these organizations will look elsewhere for solutions if nurses do not take the initiative.

Illustrations

With all the changes occurring in the health care industry, more and more nurses are considering the possibilities of becoming intrapreneurs in their organizations. And more and more organizations are recognizing the value of encouraging innovations from all employees, not just those in their research and development departments.

One example of how nurses have become intrapreneurs is the primary nursing model at Beth Israel Hospital in Boston. This program began in 1974, and demonstrates nursing's potential to provide cost-effective, high-quality care. The nursing service was given control over how staffing dollars were allocated and the authority to make decisions regarding staff deployment. During the developmental phase, nurse intrapreneurs took advantage of the decentralization process to make two changes: "(a) a change in the way care was provided to patients, that is, the development of a strong longitudinal relationship between the nurse professional and the patient; and (b) the development of strong in-unit leadership and management by nurses" (Bocchino 1991, p. 10). The focus of the changes was to improve patient care, not to specifically expand the role of nursing.

The intrapreneurial process has a long history in this institution, and it continues because innovations did not stop with a single concept. As illustrated by this primary nursing model, the role of nursing can be enhanced through attempts to improve patient care. As the environment changes, the nursing service is an integral part of the decision-making process that responds to those changes. This central role did not occur by chance; nurses within the organization have worked hard and have been assertive in their involvement in the decision-making process. Authority to make change cannot be given, it must be earned (Bocchino 1991). The same type of innovation in managed care organizations is needed and nursing needs to be assertive in developing innovative delivery modalities.

Another illustration of internal adaptation to the changing environment is the approach used by Hennepin County Medical Center (HCMC) in Minnesota to reduce dependency on agency nurses. "Seeking cost-effective, morale enhancing solutions to brittle staffing needs, the associate administrator and directors of nursing suggested a progressive two-pronged approach for reducing HCMC's dependency on temporary agency nurses. It included (a) creating an internal nursing roster program; and (b) offering financial incentives for HCMC core nursing staff to work additional hours" (Dougan, Lanigan, and Szalapski 1991, p. 128). The roster nurses program offers nurses many of the advantages of agency work, but the institution benefits because these nurses are familiar with the organization and therefore are able to function much more autonomously than temporary nurses. The core staff program provides financial incentives for nurses to work additional shifts and contributes to continuity of patient care, benefiting both the patient and the organization. This in-house response to an identified problem has enhanced the professional satisfaction of nurses in the organization, improved patient care, and been financially rewarding for the organization (Dougan, Lanigan, and Szalapski, 1991).

St. Luke's Episcopal Hospital in Houston also provides opportunities for nurse intrapreneurs through a unit-based shared governance structure. As the following discussion illustrates, a nurse plays a critical role in the organization. "The foundation of health innovative programs is the unique unit-based shared governance structure that allows the nurses on the front line to feel real ownership of their practice. This structure has evolved on some units into self-governed units. The nurse has built a culture of innovation in intrapreneuring as evidenced by the initiation of 'super units' that investigate new ways of achieving high levels of quality and productivity and the Center for Innovations in Nursing" (Curran 1991, p. 141).

The super units mentioned above are selected units that are encouraged to experiment with new ideas to influence quality and productivity. Nurses and others in these units are encouraged to abandon stereotyped, routinized thinking to be creative in envisioning a broad function for the provision of patient care (Curran 1991).

The Center for Innovations in Nursing is a support system for helping nurses conceptualize and learn about innovation. It functions as a technology transfer center where nurses can learn how to translate good ideas into actions. The culture at St. Luke's encourages nurses to take risks in trying something new and is not punitive when something fails. For nurses to become intrapreneurial requires an acceptance of failure as part of the process; if an idea never fails, then many good ideas are not being tried because of the possibility of failure (Curran 1991).

As the health care industry becomes increasingly competitive for scarce resources, organizations are becoming more interested in improving their cost position and service quality. The key to the success of these efforts is employee involvement in identifying and implementing innovations. The focus is on getting employees to discover how things can be done better in the organization.

Entrepreneurial Nursing Opportunities

Concept of Entrepreneurship

An entrepreneur has been defined by Webster (1983) as "one who organizes and directs a business undertaking, assuming the risk for the sake of the profit" (p. 608). Drucker (1985) expanded and elaborated on this definition of an entrepreneur by emphasizing the necessity of being innovative and creative in identifying and assuming the risks associated with a business undertaking. To be successful, Drucker maintained that "the entrepreneur always searches for change, responds to it, and exploits it as an opportunity" (p. 28). Alteratively, Vogel and Doleysh (1988) viewed an entrepreneur as "an individual who assumes the total responsibility and risk for discovering or creating unique opportunities to use personal talents, skills, and energy, and who employs a strategic planning process to transform that opportunity into a marketable service or product" (p. 4). As these definitions illustrate, an individual functioning as an entrepreneur must be willing and able to assume risk in creatively converting change into opportunity.

Entrepreneuring Nursing Opportunities

Although entrepreneuring is currently not widespread among nurses, the number and types of nurse-run businesses are increasing (Vogel and Doleysh 1988). Because the nursing profession historically has not educated its members to be business people, the tools necessary to be successful in business endeavors are often poorly understood and developed. The recent move toward establishing independent and private nursing practices, an undertaking closely associated with entrepreneuring, is placing increasing pressures on the profession to develop and sharpen nurses' business skills. Educational and market emphasis is beginning to change perceptions of nursing from dependent, subservient employees to autonomous decision makers capable of self-direction in providing services and managing the care of their clients (Aydelotte 1990). Independent nursing practices are not abundant in the market today, but there are a number of successful practices reported in the literature and a number of publications are available to help nurses develop their skills as entrepreneurs (Aydelotte 1988; Batra 1991; Dayani and Holtmeier 1984; Ethridge 1991; Hardy and Hope 1988; Kinlein 1977; Vogel and Doleysh 1988). The entrepreneurial role of the nurse is expected to expand rapidly in the future, as funding sources and direct reimbursement become more available and as the market places increasing emphasis on cost-effective service delivery.

As nursing expands its entrepreneurial roles in the health care industry, a variety of issues, problems, and barriers will need to be addressed and resolved. Some of these impediments are external, erected by regulations, institutions, and communities; others are internal, resulting from personal limitations. Regardless of their source, these obstacles to successful adoption of entrepreneurial roles must be identified and overcome before nursing and nurses can realize their full potential in the future health care system.

A major issue that must be addressed involves the determination of the appropriateness and acceptability of nursing entrepreneurship. "First are problems of the acceptance of private practice nurses by other nurses, other professionals, and the public. Is it appropriate for nurses to engage in this type of practice and run their own businesses? If a nurse engages in such practice, what are the regulatory and control mechanisms that should be in place? What is a reasonable remuneration for such services? Is making a profit acceptable? How does the nurse relate to other sectors of the health care delivery system?" (Aydelotte 1990, p. 195). These issues all influence the development of the independent practice of nursing and require the profession to develop a formal position on them, since they also involve ethical and legal considerations. To succeed in developing an independent practice, not only must the individual nurse be comfortable with the activity, but the public must also be comfortable with the nurse undertaking this role. To improve public acceptance, nursing must market the independent role positively and aggressively.

In addition to these external issues, internal barriers also exist. "The lack of adequate preparation to conduct business, the inability to take risks, and the failure to recognize and seize opportunities are barriers which exist within nurses themselves" (Aydelotte 1990, p. 195). In an educational process that encourages conformity and conservatism, innovation, creativity, and risk assumption are usually not rewarded. Consequently, nurses are often ill prepared to tolerate the risk and ambiguity necessary in undertaking entrepreneurial endeavors.

To be successful, independent nursing practices require business knowledge and skills and political acumen. ''Business skill involves the abilities to conduct a marketing analysis, design a benefit package or service to fit the analysis, establish reasonable fees, negotiate contracts, write a business plan, raise venture capital, make use of available resources, and secure support and acceptance of the venture. Political acumen is also necessary to convince others of the soundness of the proposal and to build coalitions for support'' (Aydelotte 1990, p. 197). The technical skills of organizing and operating a business can be learned in a variety of educational modes; the political acumen is more difficult to teach and involves identifying the power structure in the community and developing the ability to access powerful individuals. An entrepreneurial nurse must be willing to assume financial risk, adapt to and excel under uncertainty, be comfortable assuming multiple roles, be able to deal with failure and success, and be self-motivating (Carlson 1989). The nurse entrepreneur is responsible and accountable for the nursing practice and must be willing to assume the responsibility for identifying the boundaries of practice and for challenging those boundaries.

Practice Autonomy

As the health care system changes, opportunities are being created for nursing to develop more practice autonomy and control. Practice autonomy enables nurses to gain control over how nursing is practiced and to assume full responsibility and accountability in managing and providing care to clients. Practice autonomy and control are increasingly important as nursing strives to enhance its professional practice environment. In the nursing literature (Batey and Lewis 1982; Cassidy, Gautreaux and Heller 1985; LaBar and McKibbin 1986), six principal characteristics are identified as affecting the autonomy of nursing practice.

1. locus of decision making—the more decentralized decision making, the more autonomous the practice
2. amount of nursing involvement in case management—the greater nursing involvement, the more practice control achieved
3. organization of care delivery—the more independent the organization, the more autonomous the practice
4. ownership of nursing service business—nurse ownership enables greater management control and autonomy
5. nurse employment status—salaried employees are less autonomous
6. size of nursing service business—the more impact a business has on the system, the more practice control it can exert.

The goal of practice autonomy is to create an environment to maximize nursing's ability to identify and implement nursing therapies and interventions in caring for clients. The nursing profession is striving to gain more autonomous control over nursing practice. To achieve this, nursing and nurses must recognize that the resource constraints facing the health care industry are forcing all participants to develop more business orientations and to document the impact their activities and interventions have on the functioning of the health care industry (Cassidy, Gautreaux, and Heller 1985). To be successful, nurses must be able to demonstrate that the services they provide are not only beneficial to the client, but that they are the most cost-effective method for achieving those benefits. As nurses and nursing organizations attempt to convince managed care organizations to use them as independent providers of health care to members, they will need to be able to demonstrate the cost-effectiveness and value of those services.

Organizational Models for Entrepreneurs

While the current managed care environment increases the roles of nurses inside institutions and organizations, it also creates independent roles for nurses outside these entities. To fulfill these independent roles, various methods of structuring business entities are evolving. LaBar and McKibbin (1986) identified six possible organizational arrangements for the delivery of nursing services.

- Model A: nursing service company providing organized nursing services to institutions and agencies
- Model B: organized nursing service as an affiliate of an existing hospital
- Model C: community-based nursing center
- Model D: nursing center directed toward a specific phenomenon
- Model E: independent nursing practice
- Model F: private case management service.

These various business models enable nurses to enter directly into service agreements with managed care organizations to provide or coordinate a full spectrum of health care services. These organizational structures provide varying degrees of autonomy and practice control, but all provide opportunities for nursing to assume greater responsibility and accountability for the delivery of nursing services to clients.

Model A. The nursing service company, or nursing service organization (NSO), is a business entity that contracts with an agency or with multiple agencies (hospitals, nursing homes, home health agencies, HMOs, PPOs, clinics, etc.) to provide a complete and comprehensive set of nursing services for the agency rather than selling its services directly to clients. The services provided can encompass the full range of nursing services or can be limited to a specific type of nursing service (gerontological, psychiatric, case management, etc.). To maximize professional control, this business entity should be nurse-owned and nurse-managed. The NSO receives payment directly from the agency with which it has a contract. The basis for payment can be capitation, fee-for-service, episode of illness, or diagnosis-related group. Typically, the nurses in the NSO are salaried, although various profit-sharing plans and other incentive arrangements may exist if it is a tax-exempt organization (LaBar and McKibbin 1986). In order to establish an NSO, substantial capital investments are necessary to meet developmental and initial operating costs and the nurses involved will need to have a good understanding of business. "Appropriate content includes legal, accounting, and insurance services; capitalization and sources of venture capital; management of operations; marketing and public relations; and staff, physical facilities, and equipment requirements" (LaBar and McKibbin 1986, p. 8). These content areas are not unique to the NSO model; they are critical areas in all six nursing practice models and reflect minimum business skills required to achieve practice autonomy.

Model B.   In this model, the nursing service is organized as a subsidiary of, or an autonomous unit affiliated with, a particular existing parent organization. Members of the nursing service unit operate with a high degree of independence and self-direction. The central focus point of this unit is the provision of nursing services, although the unit typically assumes responsibility for securing and providing other needed services and therapies. The emphasis is on continuity of care, so members of the unit often interact with the clients at home and in the parent organization, as well as directly in the unit facility. Payment for services provided is the responsibility of the sponsoring organization since, currently, third-party reimbursement plans do not pay directly for nursing services; the nurses are salaried employees (LaBar and McKibbin 1986). Because the nursing unit remains under the protection of the parent organization, the financial resources required by nurses are reduced, but so is the autonomy of the nursing practice.

Model C.   "The community-based nursing center provides nursing and referral services to an identifiable population of families, such as families of students at a university, employee families of a specific company, and members of a labor union. The emphasis of the community-based nursing center is on monitoring health and wellness as opposed to treating disease and pathology. The center relies heavily on referral arrangements and the use of local resources to supplement its program of care'' (LaBar and McKibbin 1986, p. 10). The center is usually affiliated with the organization or entity whose population it serves, and the organization provides financial and administrative support for the center; the nurses are salaried employees. The nurse director, however, is responsible for the successful operations of the center. Consequently, he or she must be very competent in determining the population's needs, managing the operations of the center, marketing the services provided, and establishing appropriate referral linkages (LaBar and McKibbin 1986). The nurse director must be creative and innovative in designing the operations of the practice. Although the center is affiliated with another organization, it usually is held responsible for the financial success of services provided.

Model D.   The business structure of a nursing center directed toward a specific phenomenon can vary from a free-standing unit, to one that is closely affiliated with an existing organization, to a physical unit within an existing organization. ''The emphasis of the nursing center directed toward a specific phenomenon is on the breadth of care and comprehensiveness of services for one nursing phenomenon, rather than on the setting for service delivery or the structure of the business'' (LaBar and McKibbin 1986, p. 11). The major services delivered by the center are nursing, although multidisciplinary teams may be used to care for the clients. Payment for services depends on the business structure of the organization and the nurses may be salaried employees or owners of the business (LaBar and McKibbin 1986).

Model E.   An independent nursing practice is ''a private nursing business of one or more nurse practitioners serving individual clients in an outpatient or private-office setting. Clients are provided nursing therapy on an appointment basis, and referrals to other providers or other community agencies are made as necessary'' (LaBar and McKibbin 1986, p.12). Participants in the independent nursing practice sell their services directly to clients and the nurses are accountable to the clients for the services provided. A major focus of this structure is the provision of primary care services, including the assessment, arrangement, and coordination of care among multiple health care agencies and community resources. Payment is made directly to the practice (LaBar and McKibbin 1986). This business structure requires extensive business knowledge; management and marketing skills; and personal creativity, resourcefulness, and dedication. As a private practice entrepreneur, the nurse assumes the risk—and reaps the rewards—for the successful operation of the organization.

Model F.   The structure of the private case management service is very similar to that of an independent nursing practice. The major difference is that "instead of providing care directly to clients, practitioners offer case management services for clients" (LaBar and McKibbin 1986, p.13). Typically, the private case management organization contracts with another organization (such as a hospital, HMO, PPO, employer, insurance company, etc.) to provide case management services for its members. In general, the services provided through the private case management organization are: "assessment, plan development, service arrangement and coordination, monitoring, reassessment, and quality assurance" (LaBar and McKibbin 1986, p.13). These activities are provided by professional nurses and are directed at managing the overall service needs of the client in a cost-effective manner. The agency contracting for the service pays the organization directly for the services provided (LaBar and McKibbin 1986). This type of business structure also requires substantial business knowledge; management and marketing skills; and personal creativity, resourcefulness, and dedication. The nurse also assumes responsibility for the risks and rewards relative to the operations of this organization.

Summary.   These six models of nursing business structures provide varying degrees of practice autonomy and nursing control. The most autonomous models are the free-standing organizations in which the nurses control the organization and practice and assume financial risk for the operations. As managed care activities expand in the health care delivery system, nursing has an opportunity to expand its role in that system. As efforts are made to manage and control the provision of services through a restrictive network of health care providers, nursing can offer a cost-effective, quality alternative to the current medical model. The basic philosophy and education of nursing enables its members to manage the care provided to clients across clinical settings, increasing their value in the new health care delivery system (Holt 1990). It is critical that nurses develop their business skills to take advantage of these opportunities.

Necessary Skills

Nurses involved in entrepreneurial practices tend to exhibit a fairly consistent set of characteristics and follow a relatively congruous pattern in establishing private practices. Vogel and Doleysh (1988) identified nine characteristics of successful entrepreneurs: "1) willingness to take moderate risk, 2) self confidence and an internal locus of control, 3) determination and perseverance, 4) interpersonal skills, 5) low need for status, 6) comprehensive awareness, 7) need to control and direct,

8) physical and mental resiliency, and 9) a need for achievement" (pp. 26–27). Although these characteristics are shared, different individuals place different emphasis on each of them and approach the role of entrepreneuring differently.

Risk is defined by Webster (1983) as "the chance of injury, damage, or loss; a dangerous chance; a hazard" (p. 1565). Although the assumption of risk is an integral part of entrepreneurship, minimizing the fluctuations surrounding that risk through skill and judgment is imperative. While the elimination of risk is not possible, entrepreneurs attempt to ensure that the risk is manageable and therefore that the outcome associated with that risk is predictable (Vogel and Doleysh 1988). In minimizing risk, nurses must be well informed about the alternatives available and possess the technical skills and tools necessary to accomplish the tasks.

Successful entrepreneurs "believe in themselves, in their ideas, and in their course of action" (Vogel and Doleysh 1988, p. 27). This confidence in their own abilities enables them to assume control over situations and place a high value on personal and professional achievement and independence. This confidence also enables the nurse entrepreneur to negotiate successfully with managed care organizations as a provider of services. "Another common trait of entrepreneurs is intrinsic belief in their own ability to affect the outcomes of their endeavors" (Vogel and Doleysh 1988, pp. 27–28). This internal locus of control is an important characteristic contributing to many entrepreneurs' dissatisfaction with the current work environment and their belief that, given the opportunity, they can manage the situation better and achieve better results. This self-confidence and internal locus of control propel the individual to consider alternatives to the status quo. These characteristics need to be supported by appropriate tools and skills to enable the nurse entrepreneur to succeed.

Determination and perseverance are important characteristics possessed by successful entrepreneurs. These two characteristics are interrelated with self-confidence in that the individuals are sure that their ideas will work and they will continue to pursue those convictions regardless of hardships, setbacks, and rejection (Vogel and Doleysh 1988). In many cases, initial failures simply increase the entrepreneurs' belief in the value of the actions they are undertaking. Nurse entrepreneurs must also possess the personal, professional, and financial resources to absorb the costs of the failures.

The ability to relate to other people is critical in the development of a successful private nursing practice, especially as the practice expands. In order for the practice to function professionally, everyone involved must be made to feel that their contributions are valuable. All participants in the practice must also appreciate the value of the other members of the practice. Fortunately, the educational process and philosophy of nursing have developed interpersonal and caring skills in most nurses (Vogel and Doleysh 1988). Nurses tend to be trained to be team players and, therefore, can interact favorably with managed care organizations.

Most successful entrepreneurs do not place much emphasis on the external evidence of success. Private practice nurses take pride in the quality of their work and the ability to develop their potential; they do not accumulate worldly goods simply to impress others (Vogel and Doleysh 1988). However, this is not to say that the successful entrepreneur is not concerned with the financial aspects of the business and with accumulating wealth. Remuneration commensurate with the value of the services provided is important in maintaining feelings of self-worth and increasing self-esteem. Seeking appropriate remuneration is also critical in convincing others of the value of the services being provided.

"The number of tasks required to keep a small business operating is astronomical. While working at the task at hand, the entrepreneur must also maintain an awareness of the needs and direction of the business in general. The task at hand must be put into perspective and its value measured against the growth and survival of the operation as a whole" (Vogel and Doleysh 1988, p. 30). The multifaceted aspect of operating a private nursing practice requires nurses to develop a wide range of skills and expertise. The nurse entrepreneur must not only have professional clinical skills, but also know accounting, negotiating, financing, management, planning, marketing, and legal and regulatory functions. To be successful, the nurse must be comfortable performing many of these functions simultaneously and be able to maintain a vision of the entire process while working with details. This requires nurses to acquire an additional set of skills to those traditionally emphasized in nursing.

In general, individuals who perform well as entrepreneurs do not function well in situations where they do not have total and complete authority over the objectives to be accomplished and the methods for achieving them (Vogel and Doleysh 1988). These entrepreneurial individuals possess a strong need to control their own destiny and direct the activities designed to fulfill that destiny. At times, this strong desire to be in control can create conflicts with the need to collaborate with others in providing services. The necessary balance between interpersonal relations and need to control can often be difficult to achieve, but nurse entrepreneurs need to develop the skills necessary to achieve this balance.

Establishing and operating a business requires abundant mental and physical energy and a willingness to work long and hard hours— forty-hour weeks are usually not sufficient (Vogel and Doleysh 1988). In order to contribute this amount of energy to their professional life, nurse entrepreneurs must derive value, both financial and intrinsic, from the effort. They must also believe that others value their accomplishments. One thing that will drain an individual's energy quickly is to be told consistently that their activities are of no value.

"Achievement is the goal of the entrepreneur. Entrepreneurs believe that this achievement is obtainable when they apply their own problem-solving strategies, in their own way, and in their own time" (Vogel and Doleysh 1988, p. 32). Often this need for achievement leads to resentment when working for other people because freedom and flexibility can be compromised.

As the previous discussion illustrates, the nine characteristics shared by entrepreneurs are interrelated and interactive. They are essential inputs into the development and operation of successful private nursing practices.

Welsh and White (1983) identified seven basic steps that consistently occur in the career path of the entrepreneur. First, it is necessary for the individual to accept the idea that entrepreneuring is a viable career option. Second, once the option is accepted as viable, the individual begins to gather information about the product or service that will form the foundation of the enterprise. Third, the information gathered is used to formulate a business concept for meeting the unmet or poorly met need identified. Fourth, a traumatic event is usually required to act as an impetus for change, stimulating the individual to implement the business concept. Fifth, the proposed business concept is tested by convincing the first customer that the service or product being offered is superior to existing alternatives. Sixth, the information generated in obtaining the initial contract is used to identify growth opportunities for the business. The seventh and final step is to expand the business significantly. Although the time involved in each step varies with each business, successful nurse entrepreneurs consistently follow this pattern of activities.

Illustrations

With all the changes occurring in the health care delivery system, more and more nurses are considering the possibility of establishing or participating in an entrepreneurial business. A number of nurse entrepreneurs have enjoyed success in a wide variety of business undertakings. Although nurses have been involved in independent nursing practice throughout the twentieth century, Lucille Kinlein is generally recognized as the individual who reintroduced and promoted the private practice concept (Aydelotte, Hardy, and Hope 1988). Since then, a number of nurses have capitalized on the changes occurring in the health care environment.

Perhaps one of the best-known examples of nurse entrepreneurship is Carondelet St. Mary's Nursing Division in the Tucson area. In this organization, the nursing division is organized as a network of nursing services designed to organize and deliver nursing services across a continuum of care in order to reduce fragmentation and increase the comprehensiveness of services. The center of this network is the professional nurse case manager who acts as a broker for the necessary services. "Managers within the network function under a professional group practice model within a professional accountability framework" (Ethridge 1991, p. 22). As a distinctive entity, the nursing HMO negotiates full-risk contracts for the provision and coordination of health care services. This organization has been successful in increasing patient satisfaction with care received, in improving job satisfaction among the nurses in the organization, and in reducing the costs of care provided, all fundamental goals of nursing (Ethridge 1991).

Another example of nurse entrepreneurs is at the Catherine McAuley Health System in Ann Arbor, Michigan, where the group of nurses "is employed by the institution and provides 24–hour coverage seven days a week for cardiothoracic surgery, which involves perioperative nursing care for 950 surgeries annually" (Schmekel 1991, p. 1223). This professional nursing group practice has demonstrated a positive impact on staff satisfaction, cost, and quality assurance. It has empowered the members to control practice and it provides an environment that is conducive to personal and professional achievement. Members of this group practice maintain close working relationships with other operating room staff to minimize tension and conflicts in the work force. Through good communication, the value of this type of organizational model has been conveyed to other providers in the system, to administration, and to members of the community (Schmekel 1991).

Another nurse entrepreneur example is Life Wise, a two-member partnership in Westerville, Ohio, now focusing on helping elderly people become as independent as possible and helping adult children cope with their aging parents. This organization provides nursing services directly to clients and bills on a fee-for-service basis for services delivered. In addition to providing nursing services directly to clients, the partners also act as consultants to retirement communities in terms of resident selection and maintenance of residents' health. According to the partners, one of the biggest obstacles they had to overcome was the public's perceptions about what nurses are and what they can do. Before opening their independent practice, they needed to reeducate the general public and other providers regarding the role of direct access to nurses in the health care delivery system (Clark and Quinn 1988).

These are only three examples of the diversity of activities and enterprises nurse entrepreneurs have established. As illustrated, the types of services are diverse and these organizations are geographically dispersed. It is possible for nurses to establish successful private practices and to expand the role of nurses in the health care delivery system. To increase their power, nurses must be willing to assume risk and be confident in their abilities.

Future Issues

As the health care industry changes and increasingly focuses on resource constraints and cost-effective health care, the opportunities for nurses to be proactive, creative, independent participants in the system expand. "The future belongs to the visionary—to those who create new configurations to respond to new demands and who have the courage to follow their vision" (Sweeney and Witt 1990, p. 296). If nursing is to take a leadership role in forging the structure of the new health care system, then nurses must initiate and implement creative practice strategies.

References

Aydelotte, M.K. 1990. Entrepreneurs: Issues and barriers to independent practice. In McCloskey J.C. and H.K. Grace (Eds.). *Current Issues in Nursing* pp. 194–198. St. Louis, MO: The C.V. Mosby Company.

Aydelotte, M.K., M.A. Hardy, and K.L. Hope, 1988. *Nurses in private practice: Characteristics, organizational arrangements, and reimbursement policy.* Kansas City, MO: American Nurses Foundation, Inc.

Batey, M.V., and F.M. Lewis. 1982. Clarifying autonomy and accountability in nursing service: Part I. *Journal of Nursing Administration* 12(9): 13–18.

Batra, C. 1991. Socializing nurses for nursing entrepreneurship roles. *Nursing & Health Care* 11(1): 35–37.

Bocchino, C.A. 1991. An interview with Joyce C. Clifford." *Nursing Economic$* 9(1): 7–17.

Boyar, D.C. and D.J. Martinson. 1990. Intrapreneurial group practice. *Nursing & Health Care* 11(1): 29–32.

Brisk, S.D. 1986. Health care in the 1990s: A buyer's market. *Hospital & Health Services Administration* 31(5): 16–28.

Carlson, L.B. 1989. *The nurse entrepreneur: A reference manual for business design.* Kansas City, MO: American Nurses Association.

Cassidy, D.A., M.L. Gautreaux, and M. Heller. 1985. *Autonomous nursing service organizations.* El Paso, TX: University of Texas at El Paso.

Clark, L., and J. Quinn. 1988. The new entrepreneurs. *Nursing & Health Care* 9(1): 7–15.

Curran, C.R. 1991. An interview with Karlene M. Kerfoot. *Nursing Economic$* 9(3): 141–147.

Dayani, E.C., and P.A. Holtmeier. 1984. Formula for success: A company of entrepreneurs. *Nursing Economic$* 2(6): 376–381.

Dougan, M.; C. Lanigan and J. Szalapski. 1991. Meeting supplemental staffing needs: An in-house approach. *Nursing Economic$* 9(2): 128–132.

Drucker, P. 1985. *Innovation and entrepreneurship: Practice and principles.* New York: Harper & Row.

Ethridge, P. 1991. A nursing HMO: Carondelet St. Mary's Experience. *Nursing Management* 22(7): 22–27.

Herron, D.G., and L. Herron. 1991. Entrepreneurial nursing as a conceptual basis for in-hospital nursing practice models. *Nursing Economic$* 9(5): 310–316.

Holt, F.M. 1990. Managed care and the clinical nurse specialist. *Clinical Nurse Specialist* 4(1): 27–29.

Kinlein, L. 1977. *Independent nursing practice with clients.* Philadelphia, PA: Lippincott Publishers.

LaBar, C., R.C. McKibbin. 1986. *New organizational models and financial arrangements for nursing services.* Kansas City, MO: American Nurses Association.

Manion, J. 1990. *Change from within: Nurse intrapreneurs as health care innovators.* Kansas City, MO: American Nurses Association.

Maraldo, P.J. 1991. The Nineties: A decade in search of meaning. *Nursing & Health Care* 11(1): 11–16.

Pinchot, G. 1985. *Intrapreneuring: Why you don't have to leave the corporation to become an entrepreneur.* New York: Harper & Row.

Schmekel, C.E. 1991. Nursing group practice: One innovative model. *Association of Operating Room Nurses Journal* 53(5): 1223–1228.

Sweeney, S.S. and K.E. Witt. 1990. Does nursing have the power to change the health care system?'' In J.C. McCloskey and H.K. Grace (Eds.). *Current issues in nursing* (pp. 283–297). St. Louis, MO: The C.V. Mosby Company.

Vogel, G., and N. Doleysh. 1988. *Entrepreneuring: A nurse's guide to starting a business.* New York: National League for Nursing.

Webster, N. 1983. *Webster's new universal unabridged dictionary.* (2d ed). Cleveland: Dorset & Baber.

Welsh, J.A., and J.F. White. 1983. *The entrepreneur's master planning guide: How to launch a successful business.* Englewood Cliffs, NJ: Prentice-Hall.

York, C. and D.L. Fecteau. 1987. Innovative models for professional nursing practice. *Nursing Economic$* 5(4): 162–167.